Clinical Problems in Basic Pharmacology

Clinical Problems in Basic Pharmacology

David W. Nierenberg, M.D.
Associate Professor of Medicine and Pharmacology
Chief, Division of Clinical Pharmacology
Dartmouth Medical School
Hanover, New Hampshire

Roger P. Smith, Ph.D.
Professor of Pharmacology and Toxicology
Dartmouth Medical School
Hanover, New Hampshire

illustrated

The C. V. Mosby Company
ST. LOUIS WASHINGTON, D.C. TORONTO 1989

MOSBY

A TRADITION OF PUBLISHING EXCELLENCE

Editor: Stephanie Bircher
Assistant editor: Anne Gunter
Project manager: Teri Merchant
Production editor: Mary Stueck
Design: Rey Umali

FIRST EDITION

Printed in the United States of America

The C.V. Mosby Company
11830 Westline Industrial Drive, St. Louis, Missouri 63146

Library of Congress Cataloging-in-Publication Data

Nierenberg, David W.
Clinical problems in basic pharmacology.

1. Pharmacology—Problems, exercises, etc. I. Smith, Roger P. (Roger Powell), 1932- . II. Title.
[DNLM: 1. Pharmacology—examination questions. 2. Pharmacology, Clinical—examination questions. QV 18 N675c]
RM301.N54 1989 615'.1'076 88-13195

C/MV/MV 9 8 7 6 5 4 3 2 1

This book is dedicated to the proposition that basic medical pharmacology is a living science that should be fun to learn, and that it should not be divorced from clinical medicine and clinical pharmacology.

DWN thanks his wife and family for their understanding and support, and Kenneth Melmon, M.D. for his wonderful introduction to the exciting blend of basic pharmacology and clinical medicine that is clinical pharmacology.

RPS thanks his wife and family and the generations of undergraduate, graduate, and medical students who collectively have taught him more than he has taught them.

PREFACE

Many of the major advances in modern medicine over the last 50 years have been in the improvement of diagnostic tests and medical therapies (e.g., modern drugs). Thus the basic medical pharmacology course, usually given in the second year of medical school, should be an exciting, relevant, and important course for all medical students.

However, many students feel that their courses are boring and irrelevant. They complain that there is an enormous amount of material to be memorized, and that this "dry" material does not seem to be relevant to their training as future physicians. Even worse, the facts memorized in the second year often seem to evaporate by the time the student begins to treat patients and encounter therapeutic problems during the third year.

We believe that introducing clinical problems during basic pharmacology courses will substantially benefit medical students—and dental, nursing, or pharmacy students as well. The problems for each chapter were written to stress several key concepts from that particular area of basic pharmacology. The 68 chapters in this book represent important areas of basic pharmacology that are common to most introductory medical pharmacology courses. Although certain pharmacology courses in specific schools may include more topics, we tried to cover those subjects that represent "core material" taught in the vast majority of courses.

The use of clinical problems (often adapted or condensed from real cases) not only demonstrates the clinical relevance of the basic science material, but also helps the student realize that problem-solving skills in pharmacology are as important as memorization of facts. In fact, patients present pharmacologic or therapeutic problems that must be solved; they do not demand a simple regurgitation of basic pharmacology facts.

Students in the second year of medical school are more sophisticated medically than is commonly believed by either students or faculty. They are quite familiar with common diseases such as cancer and hypertension; many have relatives who have had myocardial infarctions and strokes. Many have suffered the pain of a fractured bone, and some have undergone general anesthesia. In addition, many medical schools are beginning to introduce more clinical material into the first year of medical school, in the form of longitudinal outpatient clinics or clinical symposia. Thus, it is entirely appropriate to integrate elementary clinical material into basic science courses. In fact, it makes little sense not to do so!

We learn material best when learning is fun. As the student attempts to solve these problems, problem-solving and reference-searching skills will be developed. By comparing his or her own answers to the model answers in the book, the student will discover where he or she erred in either the approach to the problem or the integration of the factual material. Whether these problems are attempted alone, in small informal groups, or in faculty-supervised seminars, they are designed to be fun.

If these problems are discussed in seminars directed by faculty, we hope they will present an opportunity for the students and faculty to work together and develop closer personal contact than can occur with the large lectures common in most medical schools during the first 2 years.

We firmly believe that a specific, separate course in clinical pharmacology should be given in every medical school during the fourth year. The exercises in this book should not and could not take the place of such a course. However, these problems do serve to introduce some principles of clinical pharmacology into the usual second-year basic pharmacology course. Thus, the coordination and continuity between the second-year basic pharmacology course and the fourth-year clinical pharmacology course are strengthened.

It is our hope that students working through these problems will not only increase their knowledge of important facts and concepts, but also improve their problem-solving skills, and develop lifelong patterns of thinking wherein they apply scientific principles to clinical problems. If these goals can be accomplished in a manner that is fun, then this book will have served its purpose.

Suggestions and comments concerning this book are welcome, and can be sent to the authors at the Department of Pharmacology and Toxicology, Dartmouth Medical School, Hanover, NH 03756.

HOW TO USE THIS BOOK

We hope that as you attempt to solve the problems presented in this book, you will gain greater understanding of the basic pharmacology that you are studying. To benefit the most from these exercises, you should keep a few simple points in mind.

First, you should attempt these problems only after attending the appropriate lectures in that area and reading the suggested material from your standard pharmacology text. These problems are designed to reinforce the material that you have already studied. In addition, many of the problems assume you have had that material as background and will build from there.

Second, try to solve the problems yourself. If more information is needed, look it up yourself in an appropriate book. You must develop problem-solving skills and reference-searching skills for yourself. As you develop your answer, write it down.* Commit yourself, even if you are wrong. You will learn more if you force yourself to think through each question and commit yourself to a written answer before you compare it to the answers in this book.

Third, compare your answers closely to those suggested in the book. Were you approaching the problem in a similar fashion? Were you tripped up by lack of information, an illogical approach, or a simple arithmetic error? Can you approach the problem again in a new way after reading the suggested answer?

Fourth, never look at the answers without at least attempting to solve the problem in writing. Otherwise, you will deprive yourself of the chance to develop your problem-solving skills. Also, you may convince yourself that you really know the material, when in fact you are deluding yourself. Force yourself to commit to an answer on paper before you turn to look at the suggested answers.

Fifth, these questions and answers may be used by the individual student or by small groups of students together. Alternatively, these problems may be discussed in assigned groups during a pharmacology course. No matter how they are used, it is important for each student to attempt to solve the problems before he or she looks at the answers.

Four frequently used textbooks of basic pharmacology are cited in each chapter. To help the student move appropriately from the textbook chapter to these problems, we have keyed each chapter of problems to appropriate

*There is usually space directly following the questions.

chapters or pages in these texts (if such material is available). The full references are as follows:

Clark WG, Brater DC, and Johanson AR, editors: Goth's medical pharmacology, ed 12, 1988, St. Louis, The CV Mosby Company

Craig CR, and Stitzel RE, editors: Modern pharmacology, ed 2, 1986, Boston, Little Brown and Company

Gilman AG, Goodman LS, Rall TW, and Murad F, editors: The pharmacological basis of therapeutics, ed 7, 1985, New York, Macmillan Publishing Company

Katzung BG, editor: Basic and clinical pharmacology, ed 3, 1987, Norwalk, Conn, Appleton and Lange

If you have a newer edition of any of the above texts, it is likely that the page numbers will differ, although the chapter headings will remain the same. Also, appropriate reading in other standard pharmacology textbooks should be easy to find simply by comparing chapter titles.

CONTENTS

SECTION ONE

GENERAL PRINCIPLES

CHAPTER 1

INTRODUCTION TO BASIC MEDICAL PHARMACOLOGY

Related Readings

Clark et al: Chapter 1, pp. 1-2; Chapter 64, pp. 758-759
Craig and Stitzel: Chapter 1, pp. 1-5
Gilman et al: Section I, Introduction, pp. 1-2; Appendix I, pp. 1561-1562
Katzung: Chapter 1, p. 1; Chapter 4, p. 50

Key Concepts

- Differences between pharmacology, toxicology, and endocrinology
- Importance of using generic names for drugs
- Differences between prescription (legend) drugs and over-the-counter (OTC) drugs

QUESTIONS

1. You are serving on the Curriculum Committee of your medical school, and are trying to decide which courses should cover the following three topics: hydrocortisone (cortisol), ethanol, and benzene. The possible courses include: basic medical pharmacology, endocrinology, and toxicology. Which topics should be covered in each course?

2. Your father is taking hydrochlorothiazide 50 mg by mouth every morning to help control his mild essential hypertension. On a follow-up visit his blood pressure is still not adequately controlled, and his physician adds HydroDIURIL™ 50 mg by mouth each day. Two weeks later his blood pressure is still not adequately controlled, and his physician adds yet another drug, Diuril™ 500 mg by mouth each day. Is such management rational?

3. Ibuprofen is a prototype, nonsteroidal anti-inflammatory drug. In the past it was available by prescription only; it was sold in 400, 600, and 800 mg tablets with the trade name Motrin™. About 2 years ago it became available for over-the-counter (OTC) purchase in the 200 mg size, and is marketed with the trade names Medipren™, Advil™, Nuprin™, and others. Why has the FDA allowed ibuprofen 200 mg to be available over the counter, but ibuprofen 400, 600, and 800 mg tablets to be available by prescription only?

ANSWERS

1. There is no one correct answer to this question. Pharmacology, endocrinology, and toxicology all deal with the effects of biologically active elements or compounds, some of which are exogenous to the patient (xenobiotics) and some of which are synthesized by the body. There are large areas of overlap among the three disciplines.

Cortisol is a glucocorticoid hormone synthesized by the adrenal glands. Thus it is appropriately considered in endocrinology. Since it is also prescribed as a drug (in physiologic and supraphysiologic dosages), it is relevant to pharmacology. Since it can produce unwanted side effects, these could be discussed in the toxicology course, although that would be stretching the definition of toxicology.

The effects of ethanol could be relevant to endocrinology since some alcoholics have ethanol-associated endocrinologic disorders. Although its legitimate therapeutic applications are now minimal (it was formerly used to stop premature labor), it is commonly covered in pharmacology. It has adverse, toxic and lethal effects germane to toxicology, and in addition may be used to treat ingestions of toxic alcohols such as methanol.

Benzene has no therapeutic uses, but it has important toxic effects on the bone marrow. Normally functioning bone marrow is under physiologic control by several hormones (for example, erythropoietin).

Some chemical entities, such as ethanol or iron, may be appropriately discussed in all three "separate" courses.

2. Hydrochlorothiazide 50 mg by mouth each day is commonly regarded as the maximal effective adult dosage of this oral thiazide diuretic used to control mild essential hypertension. Many patients are controlled by 25 mg daily. If good control of hypertension is not achieved by 50 mg per day, either another drug can be tried or another antihypertensive drug is added to the regimen.

It makes no sense to add HydroDIURIL™. If you look up this drug in a book that indexes drugs by both generic and trade names (for example, the Physician's Desk Reference or Facts and Comparisons), you will find that HydroDIURIL™ is a brand name for hydrochlorothiazide, the same drug he is taking already. Nor does it make any sense to add Diuril™, which turns out to be chlorothiazide. Chlorothiazide is in the same therapeutic class as hydrochlorothiazide (thiazide diuretics), and offers no added benefit in a patient already taking another thiazide diuretic. Thus it is very important to know drugs by their generic names, their trade names, and their drug classes. At least it is not necessary to learn drugs by their actual chemical names.

Pharmaceutical companies can assign their own trade (proprietary) names to the drugs they manufacture, but the generic (nonproprietary) names used in the United States are assigned and approved by an official organization called the United States Adopted Names (USAN) Council, which is sponsored by the American Medical Association, the American Pharmaceutical Association, and the US Pharmacopeial Convention, in cooperation with the pharmaceutical manufacturers. Once the official USAN is adopted, that is the name that should be used to refer to a drug. If you are a student from Great Britain or Canada, you will note that some of the generic names differ between countries. For example, the opioid with the trade name Demerol™ has the generic name meperidine in the United States, and the generic name pethidine in Canada or Great Britain.

3. The FDA decides whether or not a given drug will require a prescription on the basis of whether or not the drug can be labeled in such a way that it can be used safely by the general public. We may therefore infer that the FDA decided that 200 mg ibuprofen tablets can be labeled in such a way that they can be used safely by the public, but tablets of 400 mg or more cannot. We are not privy to the actual data or line of reasoning that led to that decision. In addition to labeling concerns, the FDA also considers the abuse potential of all drugs that are considered for over-the-counter (OTC) sale.

CHAPTER 2

PHARMACEUTICAL ISSUES

Related Readings

Clark et al: Not helpful for these problems
Craig and Stitzel: Not helpful for these problems
Gilman et al: Appendix I, pp. 1652-1653
Katzung: Chapter 69, pp. 802-806

Key Concepts

- Units of mass used in modern prescriptions
- Different salts of the same active ingredient

QUESTIONS

1. Aspirin traditionally has been sold as 5 grain (gr) tablets for adults and 1.25 grain tablets for children. A middle-aged woman with severe rheumatoid arthritis has been taking 12 adult-strength aspirin tablets each day and has acheived good relief of pain and stiffness. However, her supermarket now carries a brand of aspirin that has 80 or 325 mg per tablet. How should she switch her dosage to keep taking the same amount of aspirin each day? Which units of mass are preferable, and why?

2. Quinidine is a very useful drug to control certain types of irregular heart rhythms (arrhythmias). A patient receiving Quinora™ tablets (300 mg) to control his heart rhythm has developed mild nausea. His physician changes his prescription to Quinaglute™ Dura-Tabs™ (324 mg). The patient is confused because the names are different, and the number of milligrams is different as well. What are the pharmacologic implications of this change?

ANSWERS

1. The abbreviation "gr" stands for grains, a unit of mass in the antiquated apothecary system of weights and measures. However, aspirin (acetylsalicylic acid) tablets are often still labeled in units of grains. One grain is equivalent to 65 mg (milligrams). Thus, a tablet containing 5 grains is equal to 325 mg, and 1.25 grains equals about 80 mg. The woman should continue to take 12 adult-strength aspirin tablets each day.

When writing a prescription or reading the labels on drug bottles, the abbreviation "gr" is easily confused with "gm." Only metric (and not apothecary) units should be used today. For some reason grains continue to be used, especially in reference to aspirin, codeine, and nitroglycerin. Nevertheless, you are encouraged to use the modern accepted units of mass: grams (g or gm), milligrams (mg), and micrograms (μg). Also, when you write g (grams), mg (milligrams), and μg (micrograms) make sure your handwriting is clearly legible so as to avoid any possible confusion.

If you are prescribing medications in liquid form, the recommended unit of volume is the milliliter (ml). Older terms such as fluid ounce (fl oz) and cubic centimeter (cc) are no longer recommended. Cups, pints, and quarts are not recommended as units of measure for prescriptions either.

2. Quinidine is a weak base that is a useful drug for suppressing some types of cardiac arrhythmias. It is not available as the free base, but rather is formulated as a salt. You can tell from the name "quinidine sulfate" that it is the salt of a weak base (quinidine). The ionized forms of weak bases are cationic (positively charged), and they form salts with anions (negatively charged). The converse is true of weak acids. The active part of the salt molecule, however, is quinidine (free base). Different salts have different physico-chemical properties, such as water solubility, that may offer advantages in certain types of dosage forms.

When you look up Quinora™ in an appropriate book, such as Physician's Desk Reference or Facts and Comparisons, you find that it is a brand name for quinidine sulfate tablets, whereas Quinaglute™ is a trade name for tablets containing quinidine gluconate. Sulfate is a divalent anion, so the salt (quinidine sulfate) contains two equivalents of quinidine. Quinidine sulfate is 87% quinidine by weight. The 300 mg tablet of quinidine sulfate, therefore, is equivalent to 261 mg of quinidine base.

Gluconate is a monovalent anion and the salt contains only one equivalent of quinidine. Quinidine gluconate is 62% quinidine by weight, so the 324 mg tablet contains 200 mg of quinidine (free base). The physician switched from the sulfate to the gluconate preparation in an attempt to lessen the problem of nausea. In the process, however, the actual dosage of quinidine (free base) was altered as well.

CHAPTER 3

DOSE-RESPONSE RELATIONSHIPS

Related Readings

Clark et al: Chapter 2
Craig and Stitzel: Chapter 2
Gilman et al: Chapter 2
Katzung: Chapter 2

Key Concepts

- Semi-log dose-response curves, ceiling effect, ED_{50}, TD_{50}, therapeutic index
- Drug effectiveness, potency, safety

QUESTIONS

1. Your roommate has severe seasonal rhinitis (hay fever) and often takes a common antihistamine available over the counter. He has had to "play around" with the dosage, because he notices that larger doses work better but also make him more drowsy. Specifically, he has kept a log of his past experiences with the drug, and has noticed the following "rough" dose-response relationship:

Dose (mg)	Maximal relief from congestion (%)	Maximal sedation (%)
1	5	2
2	20	5
4	50	20
8	80	50
16	95	80
32	98	95
64	99	98

On the basis of his experience, your roommate has determined that 4 mg gives him acceptable relief from congestion with acceptable side effects. Based on his dose-response curve and therapeutic index, what do you think of his conclusion?

2. Your friend reads about a new antihistamine drug available over the counter that is said to be "more potent" than the one he usually takes. He performs an experiment similar to the one above, and finds the following correlation:

Dose (mg)	Maximal relief (%) (relative to first drug)
0.25	1
0.5	2
1	8
2	20
4	32
8	38
16	39

Which drug is more potent? Which drug is more effective? Which drug offers a better therapeutic index?

ANSWERS

1. Using a perfectly logical method, your roommate has arrived at a trade-off between benefit (relief of runny nose) and side-effect (sedation making him drowsy) that is acceptable to him. Any dose greater than 4 mg carries with it a moderate increase in benefit, but a large increase in sedation. By looking at the two dose-response curves side by side (Fig. 3-1), you will note several important points.

First, the maximal benefit achievable with this drug at any dose is defined as 100% maximal benefit, and represents that drug's "ceiling." Second, the dose that gives 50% of its maximal therapeutic effect is defined as the ED_{50}, and is 4 mg. Third, the dose that causes 50% of the maximal amount of toxicity (sedation) is about 8 mg (TD_{50}). The therapeutic ratio is defined as the ratio between the TD_{50} and the ED_{50}; thus, the therapeutic ratio is 8 mg/4 mg, or 2. The larger the therapeutic index, the "safer" the drug, if the two log dose-response curves are parallel.

Note also that Fig. 3-1 is a "semi-log" plot, with a linear scale on the y-axis, and a log scale on the x-axis. Most dose-response curves have this characteristic shape when plotted in this way, with "flat" portions at low and high doses, and a near-linear portion in the mid-dose range. (Of course, low and high doses are relative terms. For some drugs, 100 μg is a large dose, whereas for others 2 grams is a small dose.)

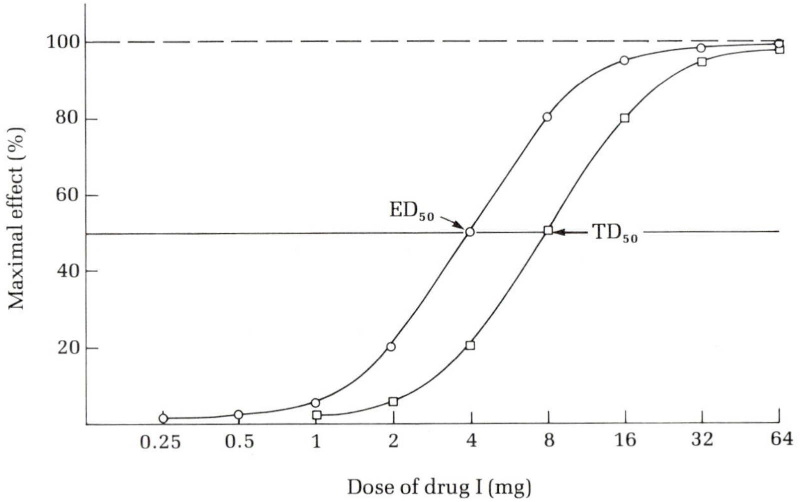

FIG. 3-1. Dose-response curves for the first antihistamine. Note that these curves represent semi-log plots. Two curves are plotted: efficacy versus dose, and toxicity versus dose.

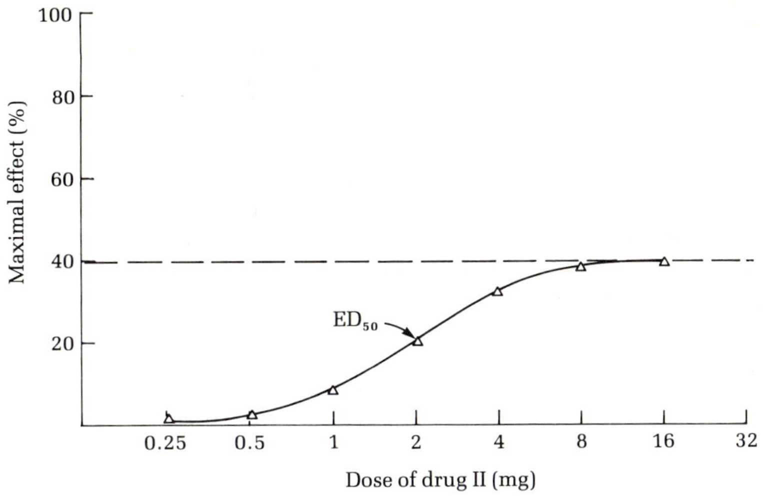

FIG. 3-2. Dose-response curve for the second (newer) antihistamine. Note that the ceiling effect (maximal efficacy) is only 40% of that obtained with the first drug. Also note that the ED_{50} for this drug occurs with a smaller dose than with the first drug.

2. From the dose-response curve of this second, newer drug (Fig. 3-2), it is clear that the maximal benefit achievable with the new drug (its ceiling effect) is only about 40% of that achievable with the older one. When both drugs are given in doses greater than 2 mg, the older drug is clearly more effective.

However, note that the ED_{50} of the new drug is 2 mg (a dose of 2 mg achieves 50% of its ceiling effect). Since its ED_{50} is lower, the new drug is by definition more "potent." You can see that discussions of "potency" and "effectiveness" can get quite confusing unless we define our terms carefully.

We do not know which drug has the better therapeutic index, because we do not know the dose-response relationship describing the toxicity of the new drug, and thus we cannot calculate the new drug's TD_{50}, therapeutic index, nor determine which drug is "safer."

CHAPTER 4

RECEPTOR THEORY

Related Readings

Clark et al: Chapter 2
Craig and Stitzel: Chapter 2
Gilman et al: Chapter 2
Katzung: Chapter 2

Key Concepts

- Dose-response curves, log dose-response curves
- Competitive inhibition, shift of dose-response curves

QUESTIONS

1. For most drugs, a low concentration of the drug (agonist) binds to a few receptors and causes a small effect. A higher concentration of the drug binds to more receptors and causes a greater effect. Eventually, when even higher concentrations of drug are achieved, the receptors are fully occupied and increased drug concentrations produce no added effect.

For example, while visiting one of your relatives in the CCU (coronary care unit), you notice that another patient has a slow heart rate (only 40 BPM). The intern begins an intravenous infusion of isoproterenol, a beta-receptor agonist meant to increase the heart rate. At an infusion rate of 10 μg/minute, the heart rate speeds up by 40 BPM. At maximal infusion rates, the heart rate speeds up by 80 BPM; no infusion rate ever accelerates the heart rate by more than 80 BPM. How would a plot of this relationship look when plotting response (ordinate) versus infusion rate (abscissa)? Now try plotting the same relationship using effect versus log infusion rate. Does this plot look familiar?

2. In some patients we wish to block an effect rather than cause one. For example, in a patient with angina (pain caused by cardiac ischemia), the usual increase in heart rate caused by activation of the sympathetic nervous system may be undesired. This increase can be prevented by giving an antagonist of beta-receptor stimulants (agonists) called propranolol hydrochloride (Inderal™). You probably know several people who take Inderal™ for this reason. If our patient in Problem A above were now placed on Inderal™, how would the two plots change?

ANSWERS

1. On a linear or log-linear plot for this patient, we have only two points: an infusion rate of 10 μg/minute causes an increase in pulse of 40 BPM, and at maximal (infinite) infusion rates, the pulse never increases by more than 80 BPM (ceiling effect). However, we can still guess the qualitative shape of each dose-response curve since we know the ED_{50}. These two curves are plotted in Fig. 4-1. Note the dramatic difference in shape of the "idealized" dose-response and log dose-response curves, even though they are describing the same dose-response relationship.

It is important to realize that the shapes of these curves are those observed in experimental animals and in patients. The mathematical models developed to describe these curves were chosen because they can accurately portray the observations made in actual laboratory situations. Both plots demonstrate that low concentrations or doses of the drug cause small effects; high doses of drug cause a "ceiling" effect, and even higher doses cause essentially no further effect; and you can find some dose that causes exactly half of the "ceiling" effect (the ED_{50}).

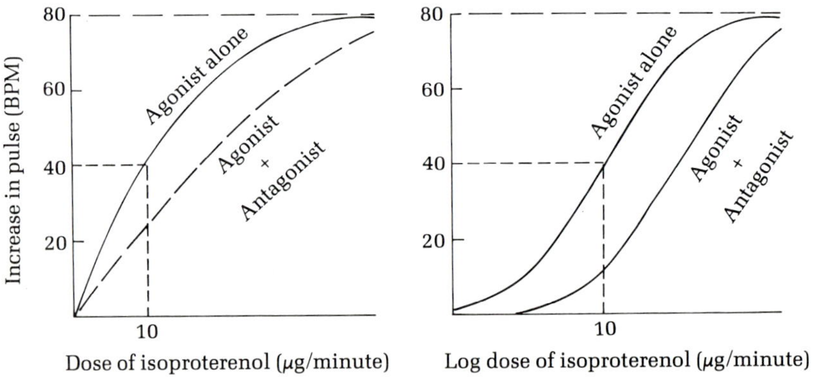

FIG. 4-1. Dose-response curves for infusions of Inderal™. Note that in the first panel, the increase in pulse is plotted against the infusion rate of Inderal™ on a linear scale. In the second panel, the increase in pulse is plotted against the log of the infusion rate. There is a dramatic difference in the shape of the two dose-response curves, even though the ED_{50} and the ceiling effect remain the same. Note how the administration of a competitive antagonist also changes the shapes of the curves. The log-dose curves bring out the parallel shift in the dose-response relationships.

2. If we have been able to plot the data in question 1, and if we had adequate data on the responses after pretreatment with Inderal™, we would see that the dose-response curves would be "shifted to the right." In the log-linear case, a parallel curve would be produced, with a higher ED_{50}. However, the maximal effect (ceiling) should be the same, since a sufficiently high dose of isoproterenol should eventually overwhelm the antagonist effect of Inderal™ (Fig. 4-1). In other words, to achieve the same effect (increase in heart rate) in the presence of a competitive antagonist, a higher dose of Inderal™ would have to be infused.

CHAPTER 5

DRUG ABSORPTION, DISTRIBUTION, AND CLEARANCE

Related Readings

Clark et al: Chapter 3
Craig and Stitzel: Chapters 3 and 6
Gilman et al: Chapter 1 (skip section on biotransformation)
Katzung: Chapter 3, Pharmacokinetics I

Key Concepts

- Drug absorption by different routes, bioavailability, C_{max}, T_{max}
- Drug redistribution, drug distribution, alpha-phase, beta-phase
- Drug clearance from plasma, rates of clearance, total clearance

QUESTIONS

1. Some drugs, such as penicillin G, are available in different formulations for administration via different routes. Different routes of administration are associated with different times to peak plasma levels (T_{max}), and different bioavailabilities (F).

Consider the new antiarrhythmic drug listed below; it is available in four different preparations:

Preparation	T_{max}	Bioavailability (%)
1 g tablet	2 hours	50
1 g sustained release tablet	4 hours	50
1 g IM	30 minutes	100
1 g IV	1 minute	100

Once in the systemic circulation, the drug is promptly metabolized by the liver and has an elimination half-life of about 2 hours. What would the curves of plasma concentration (y-axis) versus time (x-axis) look like? Why do the oral forms have lower bioavailability? In what situation would each dosage form be most useful?

2. Grand mal seizures are a common and serious problem. One of the fastest ways to terminate such seizures is to administer diazepam (Valium™) intravenously over 1 to 2 minutes. This type of administration promptly results in high serum levels of diazepam. However, diazepam controls seizures for only 15 to 30 minutes; serum levels drop off quickly, with an initial half-life of about 30 minutes. After about 2 hours, serum levels seem to stabilize and then decline much more slowly, with a half-life of about 24 hours. Hepatic metabolism is responsible for this slower phase of falling serum levels. Plot a rough graph of Cp (plasma concentration) on the y-axis versus time on the x-axis. What accounted for the rapid initial decline in Cp, if it was not hepatic clearance? What is this phase called?

Draw a rough sketch of a hydraulic model that represents the sequence of events following the intravenous administration of a lipid-soluble drug such as diazepam.

3. In your home, you have 10 fish in an aquarium with a volume of 10 gallons (40 L). Over a few days, the fish produce an increasing amount of dirt and sediment in the water. To prevent the buildup of dirt, you install a pump attached to a filter. The filter is so efficient that all water passing through it is totally "cleared" of particulate matter (100% extraction). The pump is capable of pumping at a rate of 25 ml/minute. What is the rate of clearance of dirt in this one-compartment aquarium?

Over the next few days, the amount of sediment in the water decreases, but it is still at a level that is unacceptable to you. You decide to purchase and install a second pump/filter unit that works at a rate of 50 ml/minute. What is the total rate of clearance of dirt now?

After several days the water seems much clearer. Roughly how much dirt is now in the water, compared with when you had only one pump/filter unit?

ANSWERS

1. Oral delivery forms may have lower bioavailability because of the tablet's failure to disintegrate or dissolve, less than perfect drug absorption, destruction of the drug in the stomach or intestine, removal of the drug from portal venous blood by the liver (first-pass effect), or a combination of these effects. Drugs given intravenously have, by definition, a bioavailability of 100%. Drugs given intramuscularly often have very high bioavailabilities, but take longer to be absorbed than the instantaneous intravenous push. Possible concentration versus time plots are shown in Fig. 5-1.

The intravenous drug would be most useful for rapidly terminating a dangerous arrhythmia since it achieves high levels almost instantaneously. Note the rapid peak (short T_{max}), very high maximal serum level (C_{max}), and exponential decay with a half-life of about 2 hours.

The intramuscular route would avoid subjecting the heart to a potentially dangerous intravenous bolus, and could be useful when an intravenous line has not been established. Note that the curve following intramuscular injection has a lower C_{max} and later T_{max}, but it has the same area under the curve (AUC) as that following intravenous administration. Since

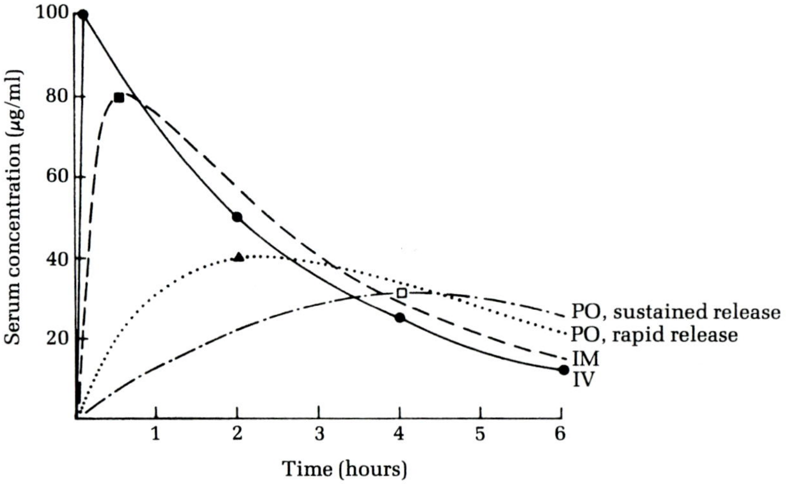

FIG. 5-1. Serum concentration-over-time curves for four different drug formulations. Note that each formulation is associated with a different T_{max} and C_{max}. Also, the two formulations with 100% bioavailability have equal areas under their curves (hard to see since time is not plotted to infinity), whereas the two formulations with 50% bioavailability also have equal areas under their curves, but only half as great as the first two formulations.

both routes have bioavailabilities of 100%, they must have equal areas under the curve.

Oral drugs are most useful for chronic outpatient use because they are easier to give or take than either intravenous or intramuscular medications. The rapidly absorbed form has a T_{max} of 2 hours, and a C_{max} that is quite a bit lower than that achieved with the parenteral forms. The total AUC is about half that achieved with the intravenous or intramuscular forms.

The sustained-release oral preparation would be best for long-term maintenance therapy with this particular drug, since the drug has a short half-life of elimination and the rapidly absorbed form would have to be given every 2 to 3 hours—very inconvenient during sleep! As you would expect, the sustained-release tablet has an even later T_{max}, and a lower value of C_{max}, but the same AUC as the other oral form.

2. The initial rapid decline in plasma concentration (Fig. 5-2) was *not* caused by elimination of diazepam from the body. Rather, the high levels of diazepam initially seen in the blood (and brain, since the drug can easily cross the blood-brain barrier and the brain has a high rate of blood flow) dropped rapidly as the drug *redistributed* itself out of the blood (and brain), and into other sites such as muscle and fat. Remember, diazepam is quite fat-soluble. This rapid redistribution of some drugs from the initial smaller "central compartment" into larger "peripheral compartments" is sometimes called the redistribution or "alpha" phase.

Eventually all of the different tissues (compartments) of the body come into equilibrium, and redistribution is complete. At that point, the serum level declines much more slowly because of actual drug elimination—in this case, primarily because of hepatic biotransformation.

A crude but interesting hydraulic model of this type of system is sketched in Fig. 5-3. In this model, the initial bolus of water is dumped into a small tank called the "central tank." Since the water is dumped in so quickly, it is unable to leave through the small drain or the larger connector pipe. Over the next few minutes, the water in the small "central tank" moves much more rapidly into the larger "peripheral tank" than out the drain, because of the larger pipe diameter. Eventually the water level in the small central tank drops until it is in equilibrium with the water level in the larger peripheral tank. At that point, water redistribution is completed. For the water level to drop any further, the central tank must wait for the

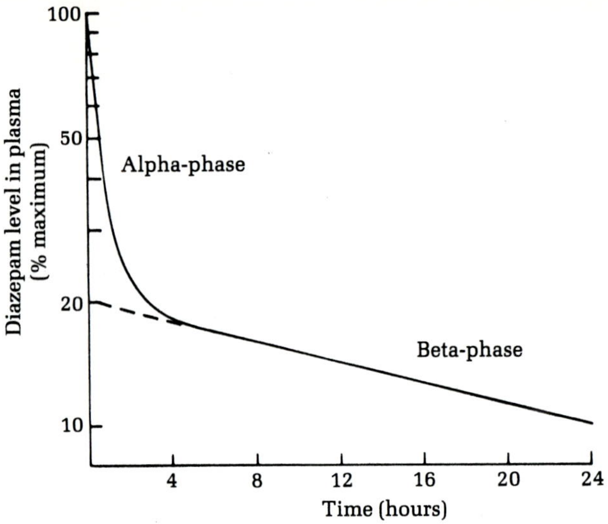

FIG. 5-2. Idealized diazepam plasma levels over time. This concentration-over-time plot is an idealized graph from a hypothetical patient. However, the "neatness" of the data does serve to emphasize several key points. Note that the intravenous dose rapidly achieves a very high plasma level that drops off quickly, with a rapid initial half-life (alpha or redistribution phase). After redistribution is completed, the decline in plasma level occurs much more slowly, with a half-life of about 24 hours (beta or elimination phase). Also note that this is a semi-log plot, revealing a first-order process of elimination.

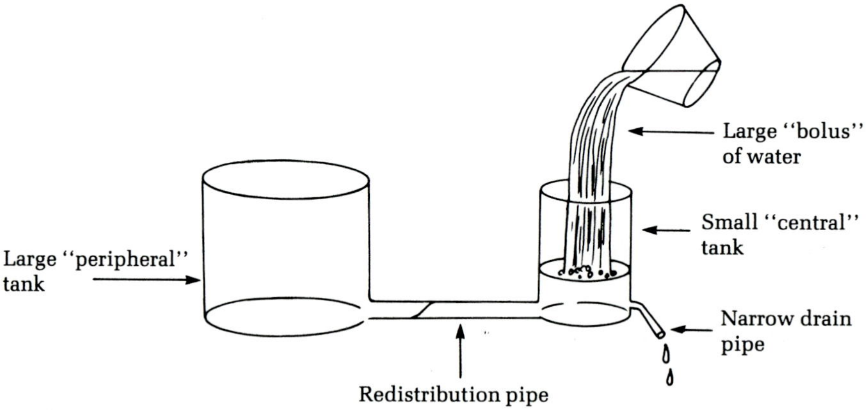

FIG. 5-3. Hydraulic representation of a two-compartment model of pharmacokinetics. Water is added rapidly to a small tank *(central compartment)* and achieves a high level. The level drops rapidly as water redistributes into the larger tank *(peripheral compartment).* This redistribution occurs more rapidly than drainage, because of relative pipe diameters. Water is slowly eliminated from the smaller (central) tank through a narrow drainpipe. As this water drains out, water levels in both tanks drop, since they remain in equilibrium with each other through their larger connecting pipe.

slow process of water elimination via the small drain pipe to begin to have its effect.

3. Since the filter is 100% efficient, the rate of clearance of dirt is equal to the rate of flow through the filter, or 25 ml/minute. When the second pump/filter unit is added at the other side of the tank, the total clearance of dirt becomes the sum of the two individual clearances (25 ml/minute + 50 ml/minute = 75 ml/minute). Remember that clearance rates are constant, are in units of ml/minute (or L/hour), and are additive.

The final level or "steady-state" concentration of sediment is inversely proportional to the total clearance. Thus, the steady-state level of sediment in an aquarium with a clearance rate of 75 ml/minute will be exactly one-third the steady-state level seen in an aquarium with a clearance rate of just 25 ml/minute. That makes sense, since the whole reason for buying the second filter and increasing the rate of clearance was to reduce the unacceptably high concentration of sediment.

Note that the rate of clearance of dirt (75 ml/minute) is constant and equal to the rate of flow of dirty water through the pump and filter. However, as the water becomes cleaner, the rate of removal of dirt (in mg/minute, for example) changes because the concentration of dirt in the water changes. It is important to realize that the rate of water clearance is constant, whereas the rate of dirt removal may change until a steady-state is reached.

CHAPTER 6

CLINICAL PHARMACOKINETICS

Related Readings

Clark et al: Chapter 3
Craig and Stitzel: Chapters 3 and 6
Gilman et al: Chapter 1 (skip section on biotransformation)
Katzung: Chapter 3, Pharmacokinetics I

Key Concepts

- Volume of distribution (Vd), loading dose
- Clearance, half-life of elimination
- Steady-state level, maintenance infusion rate

QUESTIONS

1. You are the caretaker at the public swimming pool and are responsible for the maintenance of the 100 L wading pool. Your supervisor instructs you to add enough of a bactericidal chemical to bring the final concentration to 16 mg/L. How much should you add?

2. After adding the correct amount, you notice that you have added the wrong chemical, a fungicide, which is not supposed to be in the wading pool. The wading pool is attached to a pump/filter that can operate at either 1 L/minute or 5 L/minute; the filter can totally extract both the bactericide and the fungicide. Which pump speed will clear the chemical faster? How long will it take to reduce the concentration of the fungicide to 2 mg/L, the safe limit for children?

3. After you have cleared the pool of the fungicide, you add enough of the bactericide to bring its concentration to the desired level of 16 mg/L. You set the pump/filter to run at 1 L/minute, its most economical speed. You would like to keep the wading pool operating with a constant level (16 mg/L) of the bactericide. How rapidly would you have to drip the bactericide into the wading pool to keep the level constant at 16 mg/L, assuming that the pump/filter unit operates continuously?

ANSWERS

1. To calculate the loading dose (LD) necessary, you must remember that the dose of chemical needed is equal to the volume of the tank (Vd) times the desired concentration in the water (Cw). In other words, LD = Vd × Cw. In this situation, LD = (100 L) × (16 mg/L) = 1600 mg = 1.6 g.

2. The pump-filter unit set at 5 L/minute will "clear" the water of both chemicals faster. Therefore, since we want to clear the pool as quickly as possible, we would leave the pump-filter set at 5 L/minute. As the pump-filter removes (clears) both chemicals from the water, it is returning "cleared water" back to the pool. This process dilutes each chemical's concentration in the pool. As the chemical's concentration in the pool falls, lower concentrations are passing through the pump-filter, and thus less of the chemical can be removed per unit of time. The rate of clearance of the water, however, remains the same (5 L/minute).

In addition, the time it takes to remove half of the chemical from the pool (elimination half-life) also remains constant. To drop from 16 to 8 mg/L would take one half-life; from 8 to 4 mg/L another half-life; and from 4 to 2 mg/L, still a third half-life. Thus, we better keep the filter running for at least three half-lives to reduce the level from 16 to 2 mg/L.

Now the question is how long is the half-life? We know that the half-life is proportional to the volume (a bigger pool takes longer to clear half the chemical from the water), and inversely proportional to the flow rate through the filter (the larger the pump/filter rate, the shorter the half-life). The equation for this is: half-life = $t_{1/2}$ = (0.693)(Vd)/(Cl). In this case, half-life = (0.693)(100 L)/(5 L/minute) = 14 minutes (approximately). Thus, it would take 3 × 14 = 42 minutes for the level to drop from 16 mg/L to 2 mg/L.

3. When a steady-state is finally reached, it must be true that you are adding exactly as much of the chemical (per minute) to the water as you are removing (clearing) from the water. The rate of removal of the chemical equals the product of the clearance and the concentration at steady state (rate of removal = Cl × Cpss). Thus, the rate of removal = (1 L/minute) × (16 mg/L) = 16 mg/minute. At that rate of the chemical's removal, you need to infuse an additional amount of the chemical into the pool at a rate of 16 mg/minute. Of course, if you continued to use the pump-filter unit at 5 L/minute, you would not only require more electricity, you would require 5 × 16 = 80 mg/minute of the chemical to keep up with the increased rate of removal caused by the increased rate of water clearance.

CHAPTER 7

DRUG BIOTRANSFORMATION I

Related Readings

Clark et al: Chapter 4
Craig and Stitzel: Chapter 4
Gilman et al: Chapter 1, pp. 13-21
Katzung: Chapter 3, Pharmacokinetics II

Key Concepts

- Reasons for and importance of biotransformation reactions
- Phase I reactions, Phase II reactions, active and inactive drug metabolites

QUESTIONS

1. Before trying to learn the intricate pathways of drug biotransformation, take a moment to think about the general purpose of the system. What quality must most drugs possess to be pharmacologically active? How does this property relate to drug clearance? What is the relationship between drug biotransformation and renal excretion in a general sense?

2. Some drugs may be metabolized by Phase I reactions, others by Phase II reactions, and still others by both reactions (in either order). Let us consider a common drug such as diazepam. Most of you are familiar with this "Top Ten" drug, better known as Valium™. Look up the structure of this drug. Does it appear to be a good candidate for renal excretion? If not, how is it initially metabolized? What type of reactions are involved? Are the metabolites pharmacologically active? What happens next? What is the ultimate fate of the metabolites? Are there any patients in whom Phase I reactions may be very slow, but Phase II reactions relatively normal? If so, what type of benzodiazepine drug might be more predictable to use in such patients than a drug like diazepam?

ANSWERS

1. Most pharmacologically active drugs are lipid-soluble, weak electrolytes. Since they must cross several cell membranes to be absorbed and distributed to their sites of action, this physicochemical characteristic is not at all surprising.

However, if such drugs are excreted into the urine via glomerular filtration, they will very likely be passively reabsorbed in the distal tubules and collecting system because of their ability to cross membranes. This passive reabsorption decreases their net renal clearance. In other words, most drugs with excellent lipid solubility exhibit low rates of renal clearance.

Drug biotransformation transforms the parent drug into one or more increasingly polar, water-soluble and less lipid-soluble products. These metabolites are not as efficiently reabsorbed in the renal tubules, so the net renal clearance is increased. In other words, many drugs (xenobiotics) would have much longer half-lives if they were not biotransformed into more water-soluble metabolites that are more readily excreted in the urine.

2. Diazepam has a large, fused ring structure that has few polar groups (Fig. 7-1). It is quite lipid soluble and very little is eliminated by the kidneys as unchanged drug. In fact, in a normal patient, only about 1% of the parent drug appears unchanged in the urine.

The first step in its biotransformation is a Phase I reaction (N-dealkylation), resulting in the formation of N-desmethyldiazepam, an active metabolite. This active metabolite then undergoes another Phase I reaction (ring hydroxylation) on the seventh carbon ring to form oxazepam. Once again, the metabolite is pharmacologically active; in fact, oxazepam is itself marketed as a drug (Serax™).

Oxazepam then undergoes a Phase II reaction (conjugation at the hydroxyl group to form the glucuronide) to produce an inactive metabolite, which is then excreted in the urine. Note a pattern that is commonly seen—metabolites formed by Phase I reactions have only small changes made to the molecule and may remain pharmacologically active, whereas metabolites formed by Phase II reactions have undergone much more extreme biochemical changes and are often pharmacologically inactive.

Certain types of patients may have slower than normal Phase I reactions because of liver injury (for example, severe hepatitis or cirrhosis) or an inherited defect in the enzyme systems. Other reasons for impaired Phase I reactions include the coadministration of other drugs such as cimetidine. It is interesting that even in patients with slowed Phase I reactions, Phase II reactions often proceed relatively unimpaired. In such patients, drugs like oxazepam might be preferable since they are inactivated by Phase II reactions and would not accumulate even if Phase I reactions were compromised.

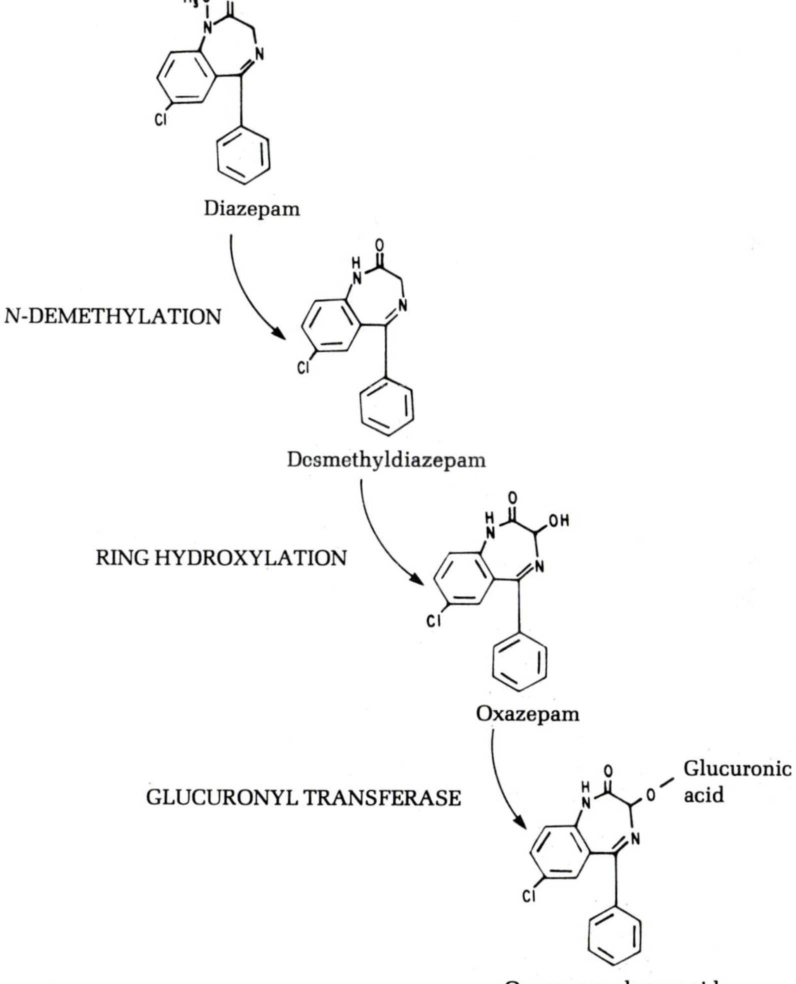

FIG. 7-1. Metabolism of diazepam. The first two reactions (N-demethylation and ring hydroxylation) are "small" changes made to the parent drug, so-called Phase I reactions. Both of the resulting drug metabolites are active pharmacologically. The third reaction mediated by glucuronyl transferase results in a "large" change to the molecule. Once the glucuronide is formed in this Phase II reaction, the metabolite is no longer pharmacologically active.

CHAPTER 8

DRUG BIOTRANSFORMATION II

Related Readings

Clark et al: Chapter 4
Craig and Stitzel: Chapter 4; Chapter 64, p. 903
Gilman et al: Chapter 1, pp. 13-21; Chapter 22, p. 575
Katzung: Chapter 3, Pharmacokinetics II

Key Concepts

- Drug metabolism to active metabolites; adverse properties of drug metabolites
- Clinical consequences of enzyme induction

QUESTIONS

1. A patient is admitted to the hospital with end-stage terminal cancer complicated by two conditions—severe bone pain (caused by cancer spreading to the bone), and moderate renal failure. The patient's physician, wishing to spare the patient as much pain as possible, prescribes a high dosage of a common and very effective narcotic (opioid) named meperidine (Demerol™). For several days this high dosage of meperidine relieves the pain, but the patient then begins to develop muscle twitches (myoclonus) and then frank generalized (grand mal) seizures. What do you think happened to this patient? (Hint: find out how meperidine is metabolized and what the properties of the metabolite are.)

2. A 24-year-old female medical student is rotating through pediatrics, and is intensely involved in the care of a young child with severe meningococcal meningitis (a severe and quite infectious type of bacterial meningitis). The infection control doctor of the hospital recommends that all medical students, doctors, and nurses who had close contact with the patient receive an oral antibiotic called rifampin, which is effective in preventing the development of meningococcal disease in anyone likely to have been exposed to it.

Several weeks later, the medical student notices that she has missed her period. Several weeks after that, a pregnancy test confirms that she is pregnant. She does not understand this, since she has been on the same low-dose estrogen birth control pills for the past few years and has never had a problem with this form of contraception. Do you have any possible suggestions as to what might have happened?

ANSWERS

1. In humans, meperidine is substantially N-demethylated to form normeperidine. Normeperidine has very weak analgesic effects, but when present in high levels, it can cause central nervous system stimulation with myoclonus or seizures. This metabolite is itself cleared from plasma primarily by renal excretion.

In this patient, the high doses of the parent drug led to production of large quantities of normeperidine. The renal clearance of normeperidine was compromised, so normeperidine accumulated in the plasma to very high levels (high rate of formation, low rate of clearance). These high levels then caused myoclonus and generalized seizures. Thus, the physician must understand the metabolism of meperidine and the properties of its metabolite to know how to use the parent drug wisely.

In such a situation, when a patient with renal failure required high doses of an opioid to relieve pain, meperidine would be a poor choice for an analgesic. Morphine would be equally effective, and its metabolites do not seem to cause similar central nervous system stimulation. This case illustrates that the choice of a drug may well depend on the properties of the metabolite rather than the properties of the parent drug!

2. Rifampin is one of several drugs that are potent inducers of hepatic microsomal (Phase I or P450) enzymes. Several different estrogens are used in various brands of birth control pills, and these estrogens usually have several pathways of metabolism. However, many of these pathways are handled by the P450 enzyme system, which can be induced by rifampin. This enzyme induction by rifampin led to accelerated catabolism of the estrogen to the point where effective blood levels were not maintained and the contraceptive effect was lost.

Such cases of undesired pregnancy caused by failure of low-dose estrogen pills have been reported in the literature. Before prescribing an enzyme inducer such as rifampin to such patients, the physician should inquire about other drugs used by the patient. This episode could have been avoided by warning the student to use another form of contraception for about 4 weeks during and after the use of rifampin. Remember, enzyme induction may occur in 3 to 7 days, but may take 2 to 4 weeks to diminish after the inducer is discontinued.

SECTION TWO

AUTONOMIC DRUGS

CHAPTER 9

REVIEW OF THE AUTONOMIC NERVOUS SYSTEM

Related Readings

Clark et al: Chapter 10
Craig and Stitzel: Chapter 10
Gilman et al: Chapter 4
Katzung: Chapter 5

Key Concepts

- Similarities and differences between the autonomic and somatic nervous systems
- Similarities and differences between the sympathetic and parasympathetic branches of the autonomic nervous system

QUESTIONS

1. It is often difficult to keep the autonomic and somatic nervous systems straight. Discuss two important ways in which both nervous systems are identical in terms of neurotransmitters and postsynaptic receptor type. Discuss several ways in which the two branches of the nervous system are quite different.

2. It is also confusing to try to understand the differences between the two branches of the autonomic nervous system. How do the two systems compare with respect to preganglionic fibers, ganglionic transmitters, and receptors in the ganglia? Similarly, compare postganglionic fibers, their neurotransmitters, and receptor types. How do the two systems compare with respect to "global function," anatomic distribution, and general importance?

ANSWERS

1. All of the autonomic and somatic nerves leaving the spinal cord (efferent fibers) are cholinergic (they synthesize, store, and release acetylcholine). For the autonomic nerves, the first synapse outside the spinal cord is in a ganglion, whereas for somatic motor nerves, the first (and only) synapse outside the spinal cord is at a motor end plate. However, there are subtle differences in the acetylcholine receptors on the postjunctional membranes.

The somatic nerves terminate at motor end plates and release acetylcholine, which crosses the synaptic cleft and stimulates nicotinic cholinergic receptors. (As you would expect from the name, nicotine mimics the effects of acetylcholine on those receptors.) When fibers of the autonomic nervous system leave the spinal cord, they terminate in ganglia rather than at motor end plates, but they also release acetylcholine. In addition, the receptors stimulated by the acetylcholine, located in autonomic ganglia, are also nicotinic in nature.

Although both types of acetylcholine receptors are called nicotinic for the same reason, we now have blocking agents that are more or less specific for nicotinic receptors located in ganglia or at the motor end plate (myoneural junction). The presence of the ganglionic synapse is one of the major differences between the autonomic and somatic nervous systems, since the latter innervates the effector organ (skeletal muscle) directly. The effector organs of the autonomic nervous system are innervated in most cases by postganglionic fibers (fibers originating in the ganglia), but an exception is the adrenal medulla.

Remember that "autonomic" does not mean the same thing as "automatic." For example, your breathing during sleep is "automatic," yet respiratory muscles are innervated by somatic motor nerves. Your heart rate is controlled by autonomic innervation, yet many people can voluntarily control their heart rates.

2. Although all preganglionic efferent fibers (from the spinal cord to the ganglia) of the autonomic nervous system are cholinergic (they synthesize and release acetylcholine), the axons of the sympathetic and parasympathetic divisions exit the central nervous system at different levels. The sympathetic division is also called the thoracolumbar outflow, since the efferent fibers exit the spinal cord at spinal levels T_1 through L_2. The efferent fibers of the parasympathetic division leave the central nervous system at the level of the cranial nerves, the cervical segments, and the sacral segments (S_2 to S_4) of the spinal cord.

The postganglionic fibers of the sympathetic nervous system tend to be longer than those of the parasympathetic nervous system. The sympathetic ganglia are usually located next to the vertebral bodies (paravertebral), whereas the ganglia of the parasympathetic system are usually found near or even within the effector organ (e.g., the intestine).

The postganglionic fibers of the parasympathetic nervous system are cholinergic, and the end organs they innervate contain muscarinic acetylcholine receptors. Muscarine mimics the effects of acetylcholine on these receptors, which are located on glands, smooth muscle, and the heart. Oddly, there are muscarinic receptors on blood vessels that are not innervated. The postganglionic fibers of the sympathetic division are almost all noradrenergic (they synthesize and release norepinephrine). The norepinephrine released can then stimulate one of several types of adrenergic receptors located on the end organs. The only exceptions to this rule are the cholinergic postganglionic sympathetic fibers to sweat glands and to vascular beds in some skeletal muscles. Not surprisingly, the end organs innervated by these sympathetic fibers are well supplied with muscarinic (acetylcholine) receptors.

With respect to "global function," the sympathetic distribution is to effectors throughout the body, whereas the parasympathetic distribution is much more limited. The sympathetic system is not essential for life, but its absence would decrease one's ability to respond to stress, especially the correlates of "flight, fright, or fight." The parasympathetic system serves mainly to conserve energy and maintain organ function.

CHAPTER 10

CHOLINERGIC TRANSMISSION

Related Readings

Clark et al: Chapters 10 and 14
Craig and Stitzel: Chapters 11 and 18
Gilman et al: Chapter 4, pp. 78-81 and p. 91; Chapter 11
Katzung: Chapter 5; Chapter 62, p. 741; Chapter 25

Key Concepts

- Effects of interruption of peripheral cholinergic transmission
- Curare: mechanism and site of action

QUESTIONS

1. A 37-year-old Vermont woman eats her dinner, which includes a large serving of peppers that she preserved herself last summer. The next morning, she notices blurred vision and double vision. As she eats breakfast, she notices that her tongue feels weak, her voice sounds funny, and she has trouble swallowing. Later in the morning she notices progressive weakness of her arms and legs, constipation, urinary retention, and reduced salivation and lacrimation. While all of these symptoms are occurring, she feels fully awake and alert. When she visits her physician, her examination is remarkable for weakness of the extraocular muscles and weakness of the tongue and extremities. She has a paralytic ileus and her bladder is quite distended. Deep tendon reflexes are diminished. Her entire sensory examination is normal. What do you think could be going on?

2. A 56-year-old painter fell off a tall ladder and broke many ribs. Since he had severe pain and difficulty breathing (because of a "flail chest"), his doctor decided to intubate the patient (put a tube into his trachea) and have a ventilator machine mechanically breathe for him. In addition, the patient received large doses of morphine to relieve the pain and reduce his anxiety. Finally, to prevent him from "fighting the ventilator," he was paralyzed with curare (tubocurarine). The plan to give repeated doses of both morphine and curare worked well until the order for the repeated doses of morphine was accidently cancelled. What do you think happened?

ANSWERS

1. This lady has probably acquired a form of botulism from eating improperly sterilized, home-preserved peppers. In this case, the bacteria (a species of *Clostridium*) probably grew in the jar and the woman ingested preformed toxin. The toxin might have been inactivated by heating before eating, but the peppers were eaten cold.

The extremely deadly botulinum toxin blocks the release of acetylcholine from all cholinergic nerves located outside the central nervous system and spinal cord. The toxin is unable to cross the blood-brain barrier. Notice that all of her symptoms can be explained by failure of acetylcholine to be released at synapses within autonomic ganglia, within end organs, or at motor end plates. Note also that cholingeric transmission within the brain (fully alert) and spinal cord (sensation intact) does not seem to be impaired.

By including this case, we do not mean to imply that botulinum toxin is used as a therapeutic or diagnostic drug (although it has been used on an investigational basis for ocular muscle disorders such as blepharospasm and strabismus). However, the properties of this toxin serve to illustrate the importance of cholinergic transmission outside the central nervous system.

Incidentally, treatment would include evacuation of bowel contents to get rid of any unabsorbed toxin, administration of horse antitoxin antiserum, and general support as needed (e.g., a mechanical ventilator to support weak or paralyzed respiratory muscles).

2. A sufficient dose of curare would produce complete flaccid paralysis by blocking the ability of acetylcholine to stimulate nicotinic receptors at the motor end plate. Interestingly, curare has considerably less effect on nicotinic receptors in autonomic ganglia, and has much less effect on muscarinic receptors in the periphery and on cholinergic receptors in the central nervous system. One reason for this selectivity is that its quaternary ammonium groups (Fig. 10-1) prevent access to the brain across the blood-brain barrier. In other words, mentation in this patient would be fully intact even though he remained paralyzed.

As the morphine wore off, this patient would be in extreme pain from

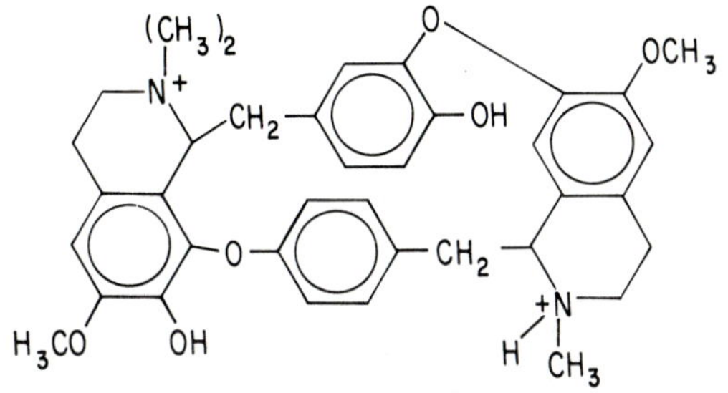

d-TUBOCURARINE

FIG. 10-1. Structure of curare. Notice that the positive charges of the quaternary ammonium groups will greatly hinder movement of the drug across the blood-brain barrier.

his injuries. In addition, he would be terribly anxious because of his sense of paralysis and pain, combined with his total inability to communicate his concerns (remember, he is fully awake and alert, but also completely paralyzed). The ventilator would add to the anxiety. Such horror stories have been reported from time to time, and you can well imagine the terrible stories told by such patients when they recover!

CHAPTER 11

MUSCARINIC RECEPTOR AGONISTS AND ANTAGONISTS

Related Readings

Clark et al: Chapters 11 and 12
Craig and Stitzel: Chapters 14 and 16
Gilman et al: Chapters 5 and 7
Katzung: Chapters 6 and 7

Key Concepts

- Direct-acting muscarinic receptor agonists: pharmacologic properties, intended effects and side effects, agents available for oral use
- Atropine: beneficial effects, mechanism of action, signs and symptoms of excess

QUESTIONS

1. An elderly woman developed difficulty urinating because of a progressive neuropathy of the parasympathetic nerves innervating the detrusor muscle of her bladder. As a result, the bladder became flaccid and distended, and the patient developed nonobstructive urinary retention. In an effort to stimulate contraction of the detrusor muscle and increase bladder tone, the physician decided to administer a parasympathomimetic agent that could be taken orally and chronically. What drug would you choose? What side effects might you anticipate?

2. A 72-year-old patient in the coronary care unit was being observed following an acute myocardial infarction. As occasionally happens, her heart rate (in sinus rhythm) fell from its usual rate of 72 BPM down to 36 BPM, and her blood pressure fell as well. In an effort to accelerate her heart rate, the intern decided to give her atropine up to a dose of 2 mg intravenously. Unfortunately, the order was given verbally and was not heard clearly, and a dose of 20 mg was given by mistake. What do you think happened to the patient?

ANSWERS

1. Any muscarinic agonist could be used to stimulate the muscarinic receptors in the detrusor muscle of the bladder, thereby increasing bladder tone and aiding bladder contraction. But since this is a chronic problem, we would like to find an agent that can be taken orally. Bethanechol chloride (Urecholine™) is the most commonly used oral muscarinic receptor agonist. It has relatively minimal effects on nicotinic receptors in either autonomic ganglia or at neuromuscular junctions.

Other possible effects include the results of stimulating the muscarinic receptors of the bronchial tree (bronchoconstriction, bronchorrhea, asthma), arterioles (vasodilatation), heart (bradycardia), gastrointestinal tract (increased gastric acid secretion, ulcer, diarrhea), skin (sweating), eyes (difficulty in visual accommodation, pupillary contraction), and salivary glands (increased salivation). In extreme cases, more severe effects such as heart block, syncope, or a precipitous fall in blood pressure may occur.

Remember that all of the above effects result from the stimulation of muscarinic receptors throughout the body. One of these effects is called the intended effect (increased bladder tone), whereas the others are called unintended effects or side effects. However, as far as the bethanechol chloride is concerned, it is just doing its job—stimulating muscarinic receptors wherever it can find them.

2. To the extent that this patient's sinus bradycardia is related to increased vagal tone at the sinoatrial node, atropine (with its ability to antagonize the effect of acetylcholine at muscarinic receptors) will help to accelerate the heart rate. Thus the use of this muscarinic antagonist makes sense, but whether it will work or not depends on whether there is any vagal effect that can be antagonized.

Atropine in a tenfold overdose will probably produce signs of dramatic muscarinic blockade throughout the body. In the eye there will be mydriasis and cycloplegia; the skin will be flushed, hot, and dry; the mouth and eyes will be dry; there may be a delirium or depression of the sensorium; the heart rate will eventually be increased; there will be urinary retention and decreased bowel sounds. Such atropine-like overdoses have been summarized by the phrase, "Mad as a hatter, red as a beet, hot as a pistol, blind as a bat, and dry as a bone."

CHAPTER 12

ANTICHOLINESTERASES

Related Readings

Clark et al: Chapter 11
Craig and Stitzel: Chapter 15
Gilman et al: Chapter 6
Katzung: Chapter 6

Key Concepts

- Myasthenia gravis: symptoms and pathophysiology, diagnostic test, desired and beneficial effects of anticholinesterases
- Miosis: beneficial effects, drugs that constrict the pupil and their mechanisms of action

QUESTIONS

1. A 26-year-old woman notices a gradual onset of sagging eyelids (ptosis) and double vision. She then notices a gradual progressive weakness of her facial and laryngeal muscles, and eventually weakness of her arms and legs as well, especially proximal muscles. She notices that her strength recovers somewhat with rest, but her muscles seem to tire quickly with minimal exertion. Her physician strongly suspects that she has myasthenia gravis, a condition associated with antibodies directed against acetylcholine receptors located in the postsynaptic membrane of the neuromuscular junction. To confirm the diagnosis, the physician decides to perform a

Tensilon™ test. What is the test? If performed, what type of beneficial and adverse effects could be anticipated?

2. Some elderly patients with glaucoma (increased intraocular pressure) have a type of glaucoma that is exacerbated when the pupil dilates (mydriasis). Several drugs are available that are quite effective in keeping the pupil small (miosis). What drugs are available to keep the pupils constricted? What are their mechanisms of action?

ANSWERS

1. If the patient actually has myasthenia gravis, an injection of edrophonium (Tensilon™) will temporarily inhibit acetylcholinesterase. This will lengthen the duration of action of the acetycholine released with each nerve impulse at the neuromuscular junction. The patient's condition will rapidly but temporarily improve, with an apparent increase in muscle strength. In nonmyasthenic patients, lingual fasiculations may occur (similar to those seen just after succinylcholine is given). Either patient might also encounter other manifestations of acetylcholine excess at both muscarinic (e.g., nausea, cramps) and nicotinic (e.g., autonomic transmission) receptors.

2. Miosis (pupillary constriction) is mediated by the parasympathetic branch of the autonomic system, whereas mydriasis (dilated pupils) is mediated by the sympathetic branch. In patients such as this one who require constricted pupils, useful topical agents would include direct muscarinic agonists such as pilocarpine, and indirectly acting anticholinesterases such as physostigmine or echothiophate. Activation of the muscarinic receptors on the sphincter irides muscle of the pupil of the eye acts to cause contraction. Pilocarpine and echothiophate are both given as eye drops in an effort to keep their muscarinic effects localized to the eye. However, both drugs can be absorbed after topical administration, resulting in systemic muscarinic and even nicotinic effects. Other drugs may be effective in glaucoma by other mechanisms of action.

CHAPTER 13

NEUROMUSCULAR BLOCKING AGENTS

Related Readings

Clark et al: Chapter 14
Craig and Stitzel: Chapter 18
Gilman et al: Chapter 11
Katzung: Chapter 7

Key Concepts

- Curare: pharmacologic actions and adverse effects
- Succinylcholine: actions and mechanism of elimination

QUESTIONS

1. A patient undergoing general anesthesia for major abdominal surgery (such as removal of the gall bladder) receives an appropriate dose of tubocurarine (curare) intravenously. Over the next few minutes, the muscles lose their tone and electrical stimulation of a peripheral nerve reveals no muscular contractions. However, the blood pressure begins to drop. What has happened?

2. An anesthesiologist needs to intubate an unconscious patient who is combative. He needs a paralyzing agent (neuromuscular blocking agent) that has a rapid onset of action (usually within 1 minute of administration) and a short duration of action (5 to 10 minutes). What drug does he choose?

He picks the appropriate drug and gives an appropriate dose intravenously. He notes transient muscle fasciculations, especially in the face and abdomen, that progress to generalized paralysis within 1 minute, thereby permitting intubation. He then notes an unexpected bradycardia. Finally, he expected that the patient would begin breathing again in 5 to 10 minutes, but after 45 minutes the patient is still completely paralyzed and requires mechanical ventilation. What happened?

ANSWERS

1. There are several possible explanations for a fall in blood pressure after a paralytic dose of curare. Although curare is relatively specific for the nicotinic receptors at the neuromuscular junction, it does have some blocking activity at the nicotinic receptors of the autonomic ganglia as well. Partial blockade of transmission at sympathetic ganglia could contribute to a fall in blood pressure. Also, relaxation of skeletal muscles could reduce resistance to blood flow through them and reduce venous return as well (decreased preload). Another important factor is that curare is one of a number of quaternary ammonium compounds and amines that directly (without antibodies) provoke the release of histamine from mast cells. The effects of histamine on vascular smooth muscles are complicated, but the overall net effect is vasodilation and a fall in blood pressure.

Just to be complete, there is another possible explanation for the drop in blood pressure. If the paralyzed patient was not properly intubated and artificially ventilated, then the subsequent severe hypoxia would rapidly result in hypotension and eventually in full cardiopulmonary arrest.

2. A drug such as succinylcholine should produce a generalized paralysis of rapid onset and brief duration (5 to 10 minutes), thus permitting intubation. Succinylcholine sometimes produces transient muscle fasciculations; this is because it depolarizes and then desensitizes the motor end plates, and finally produces paralysis. Occasionally, ganglionic effects are observed after succinylcholine is given, but they are stimulant effects rather than blocking actions. Stimulation of vagal parasympathetic ganglia can result in bradycardia, whereas stimulation of sympathetic ganglia may cause tachycardia and hypertension. Unexpectedly prolonged paralysis after a conventional dose of succinylcholine is seen in the rare patient who has inherited a deficiency of the enzyme, plasma (or pseudo) cholinesterase. In normal patients, plasma cholinesterase rapidly hydrolyzes and inactivates succinylcholine (hence the usual duration of action of 5 to 10 minutes), but in patients deficient in the enzyme the effects of the drug are greatly prolonged, sometimes with the paralysis lasting many hours.

CHAPTER 14

GANGLIONIC BLOCKING AGENTS

Related Readings

Clark et al: Chapter 13
Craig and Stitzel: Chapter 17
Gilman et al: Chapter 10
Katzung: Chapters 6 and 7

Key Concepts

- Nicotine: actions, presentation of overdose
- Drugs that block transmission in autonomic ganglia, effects of such action, confusion about drugs with similar names

QUESTIONS

1. The fatal dose of nicotine is as little as 40 mg, which is the amount of nicotine in only two cigarettes. A farmer sprayed with an insecticide containing nicotine subsequently develops central nervous system symptoms (confusion, tremors, coma, seizures), gastrointestinal effects (salivation, nausea, abdominal pain, diarrhea), muscular problems (weakness, respiratory failure), and cardiovascular problems (hypertension, arrhythmias). How do you explain these effects? Why does smoking two cigarettes result in only minor effects (e.g., tachycardia, increased blood pressure, increased alertness)?

2. A patient in the intensive care unit was supposed to receive an intravenous dose of the antibiotic, trimethoprim. The order was misread, and an intravenous infusion of another drug was started instead. When the intern next visited the patient, he was startled to find him with hypotension while lying down (which worsened while sitting up) and hesitancy when urinating. The intern was puzzled and tried to think of what drug could cause such a syndrome. What do you think it was? How do you account for the symptoms and findings? How can the intern treat the patient?

ANSWERS

1. The use of nicotine as an insecticide is now obsolete in this country, but when such sprays were on the market they were highly concentrated and very dangerous. They were responsible for numerous poisonings. Nicotine is occasionally used in modern darts to paralyze large animals. Remember that the neuromuscular junction (motor end plate) is one of the "nicotinic" sites, accounting for the weakness and respiratory failure in the farmer. Excessive stimulation by the agonist nicotine can cause a depolarizing type of blockade similar to that caused by succinylcholine.

Nicotine also has direct agonist effects on nicotinic receptors in the central nervous system, accounting for the confusion, tremors, coma and seizures. The gastrointestinal effects (salivation, nausea, abdominal pain, diarrhea) are probably caused by activation of nicotinic receptors in parasympathetic ganglia, whereas the hypertension and arrhythmias are the results of effects on sympathetic ganglia.

Because nicotine first stimulates and then blocks transmission within autonomic ganglia, the syndrome may change qualitatively as the intoxication progresses. Smoking two cigarettes results in only minor systemic effects because only a small fraction of the total nicotine content is actually inhaled and absorbed systemically, whereas the free base in the insecticide is readily absorbed through the intact skin.

2. One possible explanation for the persistent hypotension even while lying down is blockade of sympathetic ganglia with resultant decreased vasoconstriction and venoconstriction. When the patient sits up, blood pools in the legs because of loss of venous tone, and the decreased preload further exacerbates the hypotension. Another possible explanation would be infusion of a direct vasodilator and venodilator.

If you look in a book such as the Physician's Desk Reference, you will notice that the drug trimethoprim is similar in sound to the drug trimethaphan. Trimethaphan is a commonly used ganglionic blocking agent, which acts primarily within ganglia by occupying nicotinic receptor sites on the postsynaptic cells, and by stabilizing the postsynaptic membranes against the action of acetylcholine liberated from the presynaptic nerve endings. Ganglionic blockers are capable of inhibiting transmission within all ganglia, but there is little or no parasympathetic control over blood pressure. For those organs that are innervated by both divisions of the autonomic nervous system, one division or the other usually exerts the predominant tone. In the case of both the urinary bladder and the pupil of the eye, the predominant tone is parasympathetic and the results of ganglionic blockade are urinary retention and mydriasis, respectively.

Thus, you can see what happened to the patient. Trimethaphan, a ganglionic blocker, was accidently given instead of trimethoprim, an antibiotic. Treatment is rather simple. Simply turn off the infusion of trimethaphan. Since it has a short half-life of elimination, its effects will dissipate within minutes.

Unfortunately, there are many such drug pairs. For example, acetohexamide sounds like acetazolamide, and Pitressin™ sounds like Pitocin™. In one instance, a patient with severe obstructive lung disease was given a prescription for prednisone, but the prescription was accidently filled with propranolol, thus causing serious adverse results. Always be sure you are ordering exactly the right drug, do not be fooled by drugs that sound or are spelled nearly the same, and make sure your writing is clear!

CHAPTER 15

ADRENERGIC TRANSMISSION I

Related Readings

Clark et al: Chapter 10, pp. 91-99; Chapter 12, pp. 122-124
Craig and Stitzel: Chapters 11 and 41
Gilman et al: Chapter 4, pp. 81-96; Chapter 21
Katzung: Chapters 5 and 28

Key Concepts

- Norepinephrine: biosynthetic pathway and drugs that act within this pathway
- Adrenergic receptor molecular biology, inherited abnormalities

QUESTIONS

1. Several drugs are deliberately given to patients in an effort to "trick" or confuse the usual biosynthetic scheme for norepinephrine (NE). Consider the following clinical observations:

a. In patients who synthesize too much norepinephrine (e.g., pheochromocytoma), we may prescribe alpha-methyl-para-tyrosine.

b. In patients with Parkinson's disease who have a deficiency of dopamine, we may prescribe levodopa instead of dopamine.

c. In addition to prescribing levodopa, we may also prescribe an inhibitor of DOPA decarboxylase called carbidopa, which would actually decrease conversion of levodopa to dopamine.

Diagram the biosynthetic route for norepinephrine and discuss the rationale of the three drug regimens described above.

2. During a (hypothetical) student laboratory exercise, rats were given isoproterenol infusions at various infusion rates, and the increase in heart rate was recorded. Although most rats demonstrated a typical dose-response curve (what would it look like?), there was one family of rats that showed essentially no increase in heart rate. One student guessed that a certain type of receptor was missing. What type? After further testing, it appeared that the lymphocytes of this family of rats had the usual number of these receptors. In addition, these receptors had the usual affinity for ligands such as isoproterenol. What other possible genetic differences might this family of rats have? Are there any clinical situations that are similar?

ANSWERS

1. The biosynthesis of norepinephrine is outlined in Fig. 15-1. Note the small changes made at each enzymatically mediated step (tyrosine to dihydroxy-phenylalanine to dopamine to norepinephrine).

In the patient with pheochromocytoma, the alpha-methyl-p-tyrosine serves as an inhibitor of tyrosine hydroxylase. Since this is the rate-limiting enzyme in the synthesis of norepinephrine, inhibition of this enzyme by this compound will decrease the synthesis of norepinephrine. The tumor then synthesizes and releases less norepinephrine and the syndrome of paroxysmal hypertension and tachycardia is attenuated.

In the patient with Parkinson's disease, it is important to realize that the brain (or parts of it) have an insufficient amount of dopamine. However, dopamine itself does not cross the blood-brain barrier because of its hydrophilic characteristics. Therefore, its precursor, DOPA, which does penetrate

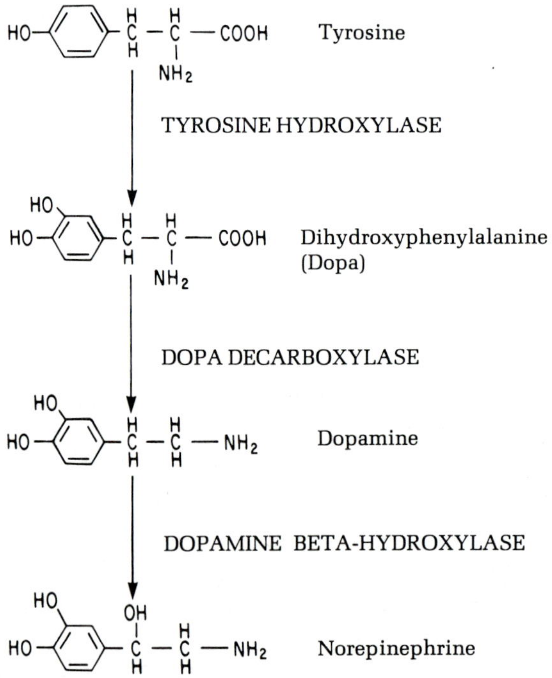

FIG. 15-1. The biosynthesis of norepinephrine. Note that each distinct step is catalyzed by a specific enzyme. The first step is the rate-limiting one.

Tyrosine

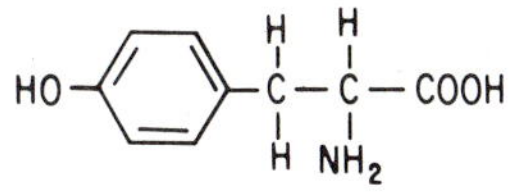

Alpha-methyl-para-tyrosine

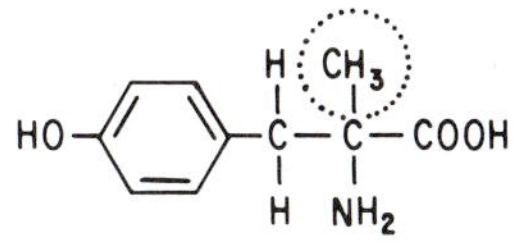

Dopa

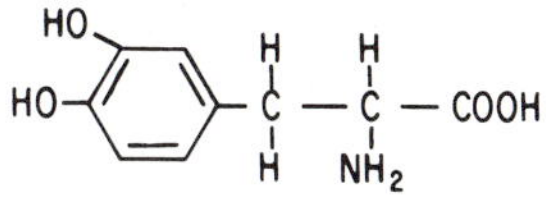

Carbidopa

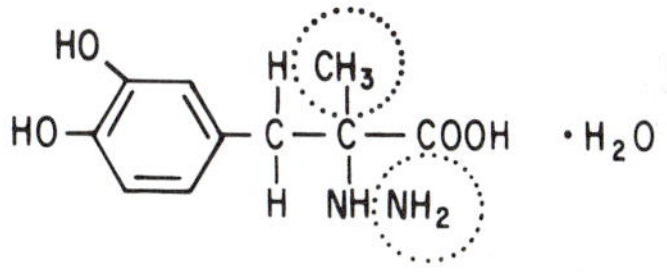

FIG. 15-2. Structures of enzyme inhibitors. Alpha-methyl-para-tyrosine is obviously very similar in structure to tyrosine, and acts to inhibit the enzyme tyrosine hydroxylase. Carbidopa is similar in structure to L-DOPA, and acts to inhibit DOPA-decarboxylase.

into the brain, must be given. DOPA decarboxylase in the brain itself then acts on DOPA to produce the needed dopamine (within the brain). Thus L-DOPA in these patients is really an inactive prodrug that must be converted to dopamine, its active metabolite.

Because DOPA decarboxylase is widely distributed throughout the body, very large doses of DOPA must be given for some of it to escape peripheral decarboxylation and get into the brain. However, most of the DOPA given to a patient is peripherally converted to dopamine, causing such systemic side effects as anorexia, nausea, vomiting, dizziness, and orthostatic hypotension. If the enzyme, DOPA decarboxylase, located outside the central nervous system, could be inhibited by a drug that did not penetrate the blood-brain barrier, then much smaller doses of L-DOPA could be given, with fewer systemic adverse effects. Carbidopa (Fig. 15-2) is a good inhibitor of DOPA decarboxylase and does not enter the brain. Thus it fits the bill nicely.

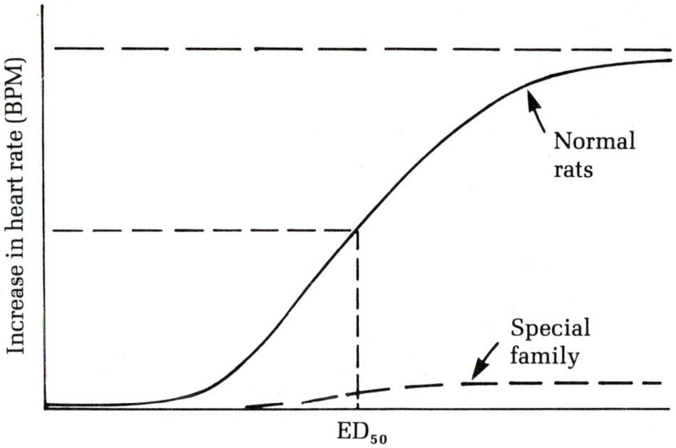

FIG. 15-3. Dose-response curves for two species of rats. In the normal rats, this semi-log plot demonstrates a typical relationship between the rate of infusion of isoproterenol and the observed increase in heart rate. In the special family of rats, the "ceiling effect" is dramatically reduced.

2. The dose-response curves seen in these two types of rats are drawn in Fig. 15-3. Notice that for the normal rats, the plotting of a semi-log dose-response curve has a characteristic shape. Isoproterenol acts by stimulating beta-1 adrenergic receptors in the heart (sinoatrial node), which has a cardio-accelerating effect. At low infusion rates of isoproterenol, there is a minimal increase in heart rate. At very high rates of infusion, there is almost no additional increase in heart rate (ceiling effect). There is some infusion rate that produces 50% of the maximal increase in heart rate, called the ED_{50}.

The abnormal rat family demonstrates a very different dose-response curve, as you can see. This failure of one strain of rats to respond to isoproterenol could have many explanations. Perhaps the rats lack beta-1 receptors, or perhaps the receptors were altered and had decreased affinity for isoproterenol. Both of these possibilities were ruled out by the results of the experiments on lymphocytes.

These beta-1 receptors on the outside of the cell are linked to adenylate cyclase on the inside of the cell by a complex regulatory protein that binds guanosine triphosphate (GTP). Recently, certain families of animals and humans have been described as having several types of defects in this regulatory protein, which result in an uncoupling of the external receptor and the internal enzyme. In humans, one such example of this would be pseudo-

pseudohypoparathyroidism, in which end organs fail to respond to PTH because of defects in this GTP-binding regulatory protein.

Although this information is new, be aware that when a drug binds to a receptor on the outside of the cell, an intricate process of transmembrane signaling begins. This binding of drug (or ligand) to drug receptor is in many cases only the beginning of the story.

CHAPTER 16

ADRENERGIC TRANSMISSION II

Related Readings

Clark et al: Chapter 25, pp. 268-270
Craig and Stitzel: Chapter 39, pp. 552-555
Gilman et al: Chapter 19, pp. 423-426
Katzung: Chapter 28

Key Concepts

- Monoamine oxidase (MAO): function, results of inhibition, role of inhibition in treatment of depression
- Adverse effects of MAO inhibitors, indirect sympathomimetic agents

QUESTIONS

1. A 25-year-old woman was diagnosed as having depression. She was given a prescription for tranylcypromine sulfate, a drug that is able to inhibit the enzyme, monoamine oxidase. Given this drug's predominant pharmacologic effect, how might it help to relieve depression?

2. The same woman has been doing well on this drug for several months and has been maintaining a special diet. One evening she goes out to dinner and eats a fondue dish prepared from a thick cheese sauce made from a very fragrant cheese. Shortly thereafter, she develops a severe pounding headache, numbness and weakness on the right side of her body, and difficulty speaking. She is brought to the emergency room, where her blood pressure is measured at 200/140 (in the past she had always been normotensive). What do you think happened? How should she be managed?

ANSWERS

1. One class of clinically useful antidepressant drugs is the monoamine oxidase inhibitors (MAO inhibitors). They are able to cross the blood-brain barrier and inhibit this enzyme in all neurons—in both central nervous system neurons as well as in peripheral sympathetic adrenergic neurons. When MAO is inhibited, neuronal concentrations of monoamines (including norepinephrine, epinephrine, and serotonin) increase, since MAO is the enzyme chiefly responsible for metabolizing intracellular monoamines.

One theory of the cause of depression involves the amine hypothesis—that there is deficient synthesis or release of norepinephrine within the central nervous system in depressed patients. It is thought that tranylcypromine increases monoamine concentrations in critical areas of the brain or brainstem, and that this effect results in its antidepressant activity.

2. As mentioned above, this drug increases the accumulation of monoamines, such as norepinephrine, in sympathetic adrenergic neurons. The resulting increase of intraneuronal levels of norepinephrine can be affected by compounds such as tyramine, which act "indirectly" to release preformed norepinephrine from sympathetic neurons. Since this woman's sympathetic neurons contain increased amounts of norepinephrine, increased amounts of norepinephrine will be released.

Ordinarily, tyramine is oxidatively deaminated in the liver after oral absorption and never reaches the systemic circulation as tyramine. In this patient, the MAO in the liver is inhibited along with the MAO in the sympathetic nerves. Thus, tyramine is not "detoxified" and it reaches the systemic circulation in its active form to provoke a hypertensive crisis.

Tyramine is a protein breakdown product that occurs in variable amounts in aged (or fermented) foods, such as some cheeses, yogurts, or wines. In this patient, the fondue sauce she consumed was made from a cheese with a high tyramine content. After the tyramine was ingested, it caused a sudden release of large quantities of norepinephrine from sympathetic neurons, creating a sympathetic crisis. Other drugs that owe at least part of their activity to tyramine-like release of preformed norepinephrine include metaraminol, amphetamine, and ephedrine. The pounding headache and neurologic symptoms were related to the abrupt hypertensive crisis.

Although the blood pressure may gradually return towards normal as the released norepinephrine is removed or metabolized, some patients must be given an antidote. Since the abrupt hypertension is caused by the stimulation of alpha-1 receptors by norepinephrine, treatment usually consists of intravenous administration of an alpha-receptor blocker, such as phentolamine. In this case, the treatment was successful and the patient's neurologic problems rapidly disappeared. These patients should be instructed about which foods to avoid, and should wear a bracelet that lists their medication and antidote.

CHAPTER 17

ADRENERGIC RECEPTOR AGONISTS

Related Readings

Clark et al: Chapter 15
Craig and Stitzel: Chapter 12
Gilman et al: Chapter 8
Katzung: Chapter 8

Key Concepts

- Use of pure alpha-receptor agonists, use of mixed alpha- and beta-receptor agonists, hemodynamic abnormalities in septic and anaphylactic shock
- Beta receptor agonists, beta-1 selective agonists, beta-2 selective agonists, treatment of cardiogenic shock, treatment of bronchospasm

QUESTIONS

1. You admit two patients to the emergency department. The first patient is suffering from *septic shock* (shock associated with a serious infection, usually bacterial) in which the primary hemodynamic findings are tachycardia, high cardiac output, and extreme arteriolar vasodilation, resulting in profound hypotension. A second patient is admitted who is also in shock after suffering a hornet sting. This type of shock is called *anaphylactic shock*, and is associated with hypotension, tachycardia or bradycardia, swollen lips and tongue (angioedema), wheezing (bronchospasm), and hives (urticaria). Discuss the following three questions for each type of shock:

1. What are your specific goals of pharmacologic intervention?
2. What type of adrenergic receptors mediate those goals?
3. Which drug (agonist) would best stimulate the receptors that should be stimulated?

2. The next night you are on call, you again admit two gravely ill patients. The first is an elderly man who has had a serious heart attack and is also in shock. This type of shock, called *cardiogenic shock*, is associated with low cardiac output, tachycardia, and extreme vasoconstriction. The second patient is admitted with acute severe bronchospasm, associated with a flare of his intermittent asthma. His blood pressure is satisfactory, but he is quite tachycardic. Again, discuss the following three questions for each patient:

1. What are your specific goals of pharmacologic intervention?
2. What type of adrenergic receptors mediate those goals?
3. Which drug (agonist) would best stimulate the receptors that should be stimulated?

ANSWERS

1. The patient in septic shock already has tachycardia, high cardiac output, extreme arteriolar vasodilatation, and profound hypotension. Goals of management would include treating the infection and correcting the primary physiologic abnormality. Therapy would begin with expanding the blood volume (by giving intravenous fluids) and treating the infection with appropriate antibiotics.

After that, vasoconstriction could be achieved by stimulating alpha-1 adrenergic receptors while avoiding stimulation of beta-1 and beta-2 receptors. Any adrenergic agonist active on beta receptors (beta-1 cardiac stimulation and beta-2 vasodilation in skeletal and heart muscle) would not be useful and might even be harmful. Relatively selective stimulation of alpha-1 adrenergic receptors could be achieved by using such drugs as phenylephrine or methoxamine. Less selective stimulation of alpha-1 receptors would be achieved by using norepinephrine.

The signs and symptoms of anaphylactic shock are caused by sudden and massive release of histamine and other autacoids. A drug is needed that will prevent further degranulation of mast cells and also counter the effects of vasodilatation and bronchospasm. Vasoconstriction is mediated by alpha-1 receptors, whereas mast cells can be stabilized by stimulation of beta-1 and/or beta-2 receptors. Bronchodilation is achieved by stimulating beta-2 receptors. Epinephrine is the drug of choice in this situation, since it is a mixed agonist with effects on alpha-1, beta-1, and beta-2 receptors. No other adrenergic agonist is nearly as effective in this role. Antihistamines have a secondary role in management, but are not the "first line" drugs of choice in life-threatening allergic reactions.

2. The patient in cardiogenic shock has a low cardiac output, tachycardia, and extreme vasoconstriction. This patient would benefit from a drug that would increase cardiac output but not cause an increase in heart rate or degree of vasoconstriction; in fact, mild vasodilatation might be beneficial. Activation of alpha-1 receptors should be carefully avoided. Isoproterenol could stimulate cardiac beta-1 receptors and peripheral beta-2 receptors, but it causes unacceptable tachycardia. Dopamine stimulates these receptors as well as peripheral dopaminergic receptors and alpha-1 receptors, which might worsen the vasoconstriction. In this patient, dobutamine might be the best drug, since it may be able to increase cardiac output (beta-1 receptors) with minimal increase in heart rate, cause mild peripheral vasodilation (beta-1 and beta-2 stimulation), and does not stimulate alpha-1 receptors.

For the asthmatic patient in bronchospasm who already has tachycardia, we want to selectively stimulate beta-2 receptors to produce bronchodilation but avoid activating beta-1 receptors in the heart, which would worsen the tachycardia already present. A drug with "selective" ability to stimulate only beta-2 receptors would be ideal. Drugs with this property include metaproterenol, albuterol, isoetharine, and terbutaline. Of these, albuterol is probably the most beta-2 selective and clinically useful.

CHAPTER 18

ADRENERGIC RECEPTOR ANTAGONISTS

Related Readings

Clark et al: Chapter 16
Craig and Stitzel: Chapter 13
Gilman et al: Chapter 9, pp. 181-203
Katzung: Chapter 9

Key Concepts

- Symptoms of pheochromocytoma, hypertensive actions of catecholamines, consequences of alpha-receptor antagonists
- Indications for beta-receptor antagonists, difference between mixed beta-1/beta-2 antagonists and "selective" beta-1 receptor antagonists

QUESTIONS

1. A 42-year-old woman experiences episodes of severe headache, palpitations, and severe hypertension. A thorough examination reveals that all symptoms are caused by a pheochromocytoma (a tumor that produces catecholamines). Before performing surgery to remove the tumor, the physician needs to control the blood pressure by counteracting the effects of the surges of norepinephrine (performing surgery without obtaining this preoperative control can cause an extreme hypertensive crisis). Which agents would be useful in this regard?

2. As a third-year student, you are working in a busy outpatient clinic and find yourself treating two interesting patients. The first is a young woman who has symptoms and laboratory findings that document severe hyperthyroidism (nervousness, diarrhea, tremor, sweating, palpitations, and tachycardia). Although a more definitive type of therapy is being ordered, you decide to treat some of the symptoms with a beta-receptor antagonist. Which one would you choose?

Your next patient has hypertension with angina—both indications for the use of a beta-blocking drug. However, his case is complicated by the presence of mild asthma. If you prescribed a beta-blocker, which one would you use in this case?

ANSWERS

1. In the patient with a pheochromocytoma, it would be best to use an alpha-1 receptor blocking drug to control the blood pressure and prevent such catastrophic events as a ruptured cerebral aneurysm. During surgery, the surgeon must manipulate the tumor, and as norepinephrine is "squeezed" out, the blood pressure may climb to very high levels (massive vasoconstriction mediated by alpha-1 receptors). Reasonable choices would include prazosin, phentolamine, phenoxybenzamine, or tolazoline. Because of its longer duration of action and oral availability, phenoxybenzamine is usually given in this situation for several weeks before surgery. During surgery, intravenous doses of phentolamine could also be given as needed to help control blood pressure surges.

Occasionally, a patient will also need to be treated with a beta-receptor blocker to blunt the tachycardia sometimes seen. Remember that the beta-blocker should be given only after the patient has been satisfactorily treated with an alpha-blocker; a beta-blocker alone may actually make the hypertension worse by preventing beta-2 mediated vasodilation but not preventing alpha-1 mediated vasoconstriction.

Also, do not forget that you have already learned about a drug that can decrease the synthesis of norepinephrine by the tumor. Alpha-methyl-para-tyrosine may also be given in this situation to inhibit tyrosine hydroxylase, the rate limiting enzyme in the synthesis of norepinephrine. Many patients with a pheochromocytoma are controlled before surgery by a combination of phenoxybenzamine and alpha-methyl-para-tyrosine.

2. The severe hyperthyroidism should be treated with either antithyroid drugs, radiation by ingestion of radioactive iodine, or surgery (subtotal thyroidectomy). However, all of these therapeutic modalities require time to work, and many of the unpleasant symptoms of hyperthyroidism (which resemble activation of the sympathetic nervous system) can persist for weeks. The connection between hyperthyroidism and activation of the sympathetic nervous system is not entirely understood. However, extensive experience with propranolol, a nonspecific beta-blocker, indicates that some of the symptoms of hyperthyroidism (e.g., tachycardia, palpitations, tremor) can be ameliorated promptly by use of this drug. Much less experience has been obtained with other beta-blockers, although several others are on the market with other FDA-approved indications. Therefore, propranolol would be the drug of choice in this situation.

For the hypertensive patient with angina, a beta-blocker (or a recently approved calcium channel blocker) could help both conditions. If a beta-blocker is chosen, a nonspecific beta-blocker would block both beta-1 and beta-2 receptors, thereby making the patient's asthma worse. Thus, a "selective" beta-1 receptor blocker such as metoprolol or atenolol would be preferable to a nonselective beta-blocker such as propranolol, nadolol, or timolol. Few agonist or antagonist drugs, however, are completely selective; therefore, it is advisable to proceed cautiously and watch for signs indicative of aggravation of the patient's asthma.

CHAPTER 19

DRUG EFFECTS ON ADRENERGIC NERVE ENDINGS

Related Readings

Clark et al: Chapter 17
Craig and Stitzel: Chapter 22, pp. 318-323
Gilman et al: Chapter 9, pp. 209-211
Katzung: Chapter 10, pp. 113-115

Key Concepts

- Reserpine: mechanism of action, consequences of amine depletion, adverse drug effects
- Guanethidine: mechanisms of action and drug interactions

QUESTIONS

1. Reserpine has proven to be an effective and inexpensive agent useful in the management of hypertension. It seems to work by decreasing cardiac output and peripheral vascular resistance, and causes little postural hypotension. However, some patients develop sedation, mental depression, parkinsonism, and mild diarrhea or cramps. Why do you think these central nervous system and gastrointestinal symptoms (adverse effects) occur?

2. A patient in your clinic has severe essential hypertension (blood pressure 240/140) that has not responded well to several drugs. One of the clinic physicians added guanethidine to his other two medications, and the blood pressure came down nicely to 150/90. How did the drug work at the neuronal level?

Several weeks later, his blood pressure abruptly climbs back to his pretreatment level; when you talk to the patient, the only change in his life has been that he has begun using one new drug, amitriptyline. Why did his blood pressure climb back to a dangerous level?

ANSWERS

1. Reserpine depletes the nerve endings' transmitter stores of norepinephrine (noradrenergic neurons), dopamine (dopaminergic neurons), or serotonin (5-HT, serotoninergic neurons) by blocking the active transport process that packages these transmitters into secretory granules. Failure of noradrenergic transmission, probably in the cerebral cortex, leads to sedation and psychiatric depression. Failure of dopaminergic transmission in the basal ganglia may lead to signs of parkinsonism. Failure of noradrenergic transmission in the intestine leads to a preponderance of parasympathetic tone with increases in gut motility, diarrhea, and cramps.

2. Guanethidine lowers blood pressure and rapidly blocks sympathetic transmission by a "local anesthetic" action on adrenergic nerve terminals. This prevents the release of norepinephrine in response to nerve action potentials. Following this, norepinephrine is slowly released from the nerve ending so the terminal is eventually depleted of its neurotransmitter. Some transmission is sustained by virtue of continued synthesis and the ability of the neuron to conserve norepinephrine by active uptake from the synaptic cleft; in addition, postsynaptic receptors may become supersensitive to norepinephrine.

However, guanethidine must be taken up by the adrenergic neurons for it to be effective. Amitriptyline, a tricyclic antidepressant drug, apparently inhibits the neuronal uptake of guanethidine. The blood pressure can rapidly rise back towards the original level; when amitriptyline is stopped, the blood pressure will drop again over 5 days or so. It is best to avoid this drug combination.

SECTION THREE

AUTACOIDS AND ANTI-INFLAMMATORY DRUGS

CHAPTER 20

HISTAMINE AGONISTS AND ANTAGONISTS

Related Readings

Clark et al: Chapters 19 and 20
Craig and Stitzel: Chapter 70
Gilman et al: Chapter 26, pp. 604-628
Katzung: Chapter 15, pp. 183-192

Key Concepts

- Systemic effects of histamine
- Actions, types of histamine receptor blocking drugs

QUESTIONS

1. A patient develops the syndrome of systemic mastocytosis. In this syndrome, there are excessive numbers of mast cells in the body that have a tendency to degranulate, releasing large amounts of histamine and other vasoactive substances. Assuming that histamine is the most important autacoid released, what symptoms would you expect the patient to manifest?

2. In an effort to treat these symptoms, you have prescribed diphenhydramine, a prototypical antihistamine compound. How does this drug work? The patient says that with this treatment he feels somewhat better, but still is quite symptomatic. What else could you try?

ANSWERS

1. A patient with mastocytosis would experience episodes of hypotension, flushing, urticaria, itching, and perhaps other symptoms caused by the episodic release of histamine. Vasodilatation would trigger a reflex tachycardia that the patient might describe as palpitations. Histamine would tend to produce bronchoconstriction, especially in asthmatic patients. Histamine could also cause increased gastric acid secretion, which could lead to activation of peptic ulcers. Increased intestinal motility might result in diarrhea and cramping.

2. Diphenhydramine is a competitive H-1 receptor blocking drug (antagonist). It would not completely control the blood pressure response to histamine, which is mediated in part through stimulation of H-2 receptors. It would tend to reverse the bronchoconstriction in normal patients, but it would not help much in the asthmatic. It should relieve the increase in gut motility and help with the hives, but the increased gastric secretions are mediated through H-2 receptors. The latter can be competitively blocked with cimetidine or ranitidine hydrochloride, both H-2 receptor blocking drugs. Such patients often benefit from simultaneous treatment with both an H-1 blocker and an H-2 blocker.

In this situation, we have better pharmacologic tools for blocking the effects of a released autacoid (histamine) than for preventing its release from mast cells in the first place.

CHAPTER 21

PROSTAGLANDINS

Related Readings

Clark et al: Chapters 22 and 31
Craig and Stitzel: Chapters 19 and 42
Gilman et al: Chapter 28 and Chapter 29, pp. 674-708
Katzung: Chapter 17 and Chapter 34, pp. 396-409

Key Concepts

- Roles of prostacyclin and thromboxane A_2
- Physiologic effects of renal prostaglandins

QUESTIONS

1. To prevent recurrent heart attacks and help treat severe angina (cardiac ischemic pain), many doctors now prescribe aspirin 80 mg (1 pediatric aspirin tablet) or 325 mg (1 adult aspirin tablet) each day. On the theory that "more is better," some patients take two tablets (650 mg) three or four times daily. Why may that not be such a good idea?

2. When nonsteroidal anti-inflammatory drugs (NSAIDs) are given to healthy patients, very few develop renal problems. However, when patients with other major medical problems such as hypotension, hemorrhage, salt depletion, heart failure or those undergoing general anesthesia receive these drugs, they may develop a number of renal syndromes, including acute renal failure (abrupt deterioration in renal function). Why are the side effects of this class of drugs apparently different in healthy and sick patients?

ANSWERS

1. The recommendation to take 80 to 325 mg of aspirin daily to prevent a second heart attack or to help control severe angina is based on the ability of aspirin to inhibit (irreversibly) the enzyme cyclooxygenase in blood platelets (Fig. 21-1). This effect prevents the synthesis of thromboxane A_2 by platelets. Since thromboxane A_2 promotes platelet aggregation and arteriolar constriction, it would be desirable to inhibit its production in these patients. This effect of aspirin is dangerous in some situations (e.g., in hemophiliacs and patients with other clotting disorders or in patients receiving intensive anticoagulant therapy). The same effect, however, may be life saving in patients at risk for a second heart attack, stroke, or thromboembolic disease.

The maximum therapeutic effect of aspirin for these indications is achieved at the low dosages recommended above. Nothing is gained by increasing the dose of aspirin; instead, much may be lost. At higher dosages and concentrations, aspirin inhibits prostacyclin (PGI_2) formation in the vascular endothelium. Since prostacyclin inhibits platelet aggregation

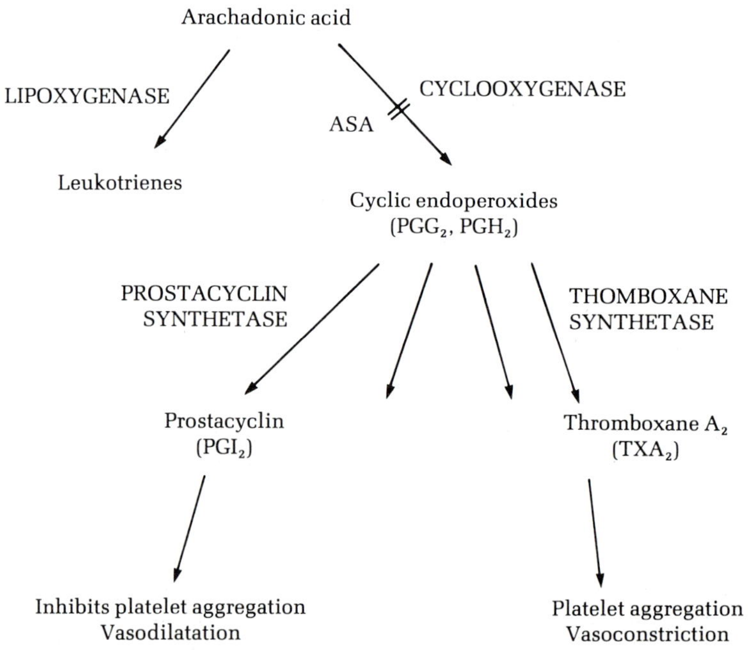

FIG. 21-1. Inhibition of cyclooxygenase by aspirin. Note especially the effects of aspirin upon production of both thromboxane A_2 and prostacyclin.

and contributes to arteriolar dilatation, we would *not* want to inhibit its production in these patients. Thus, a small dose of aspirin (which selectively inhibits thromboxane A_2 production) is more effective than a larger dose of aspirin (which inhibits the production of both thromboxane A_2 and prostacyclin).

2. Local prostaglandin production by the kidney appears to help regulate renal blood flow, renin release, and renal sodium loss. Even so, NSAID have little effect on renal function in normal humans.

However, in some patients with the medical conditions listed in this question, there may be very high venous levels of various vasoconstrictor hormones such as norepinephrine and angiotensin II. The vasodilating prostaglandins produced in the kidney may be essential in maintaining renal blood flow. If their synthesis is blocked by a NSAID, then an abrupt decrease in renal blood flow, with associated renal failure, may follow. Thus, the effects of a NSAID (or any other drug) may be quite different in healthy volunteers (who are not dependent on renal prostaglandins for adequate renal function) and in sick patients (who are very dependent on renal prostaglandins to maintain adequate renal function).

CHAPTER 22

SALICYLATES AND NONSTEROIDAL ANTI-INFLAMMATORY DRUGS (NSAID)

Related Readings

Clark et al: Chapter 31
Craig and Stitzel: Chapter 42
Gilman et al: Chapter 29, pp. 674-708
Katzung: Chapter 34, pp. 396-409

Key Concepts

- Differences in salicylate preparations, other active ingredients
- Signs and symptoms of subacute salicylate toxicity; salicylate kinetics; enhancement of renal excretion
- Different classes and properties of nonsteroidal anti-inflammatory drugs (NSAID)

QUESTIONS

1. A woman with severe rheumatoid arthritis takes 14 aspirin tablets (325 mg each) each day to control her joint pain and stiffness. This works fairly well, and her problems are minimal as long as she takes her aspirin with meals. She sees a television advertisement that claims that Alka-Seltzer™ speeds relief to the bloodstream faster than "regular aspirin tablets," and she decides to switch from aspirin tablets to Alka-Seltzer tablets. Will this switch result in faster absorption? Will it alter overall bioavailability or the steady-state plasma salicylate level? Will it change the extent of gastric damage? What other ingredients are in Alka-Seltzer™? What would be the difference in cost per month of treatment?

2. An elderly woman becomes confused about her medications, and begins to take 20 aspirin tablets per day instead of her usual seven. Over several days she becomes more agitated and confused, and she develops a ringing in her ears, nausea, and vomiting. She is brought to the emergency room where she has a temperature of 103° F, a bounding pulse of 130, a blood pressure of 95/65 mm Hg, a respiratory rate of 36 breaths per minute. Her skin is flushed and moist. There is little urine in her bladder. Her laboratory values reveal a combination of respiratory alkalosis and metabolic acidosis. What accounts for these symptoms? How can you help her eliminate the salicylate from her body more quickly?

3. The increasing number of NSAID approved by the FDA makes their rational use quite confusing. Some drugs are advertised for their analgesic effects, others for their effects on arthritis, and still others for their ability to treat both arthritis and other types of pain. What are the important differences among the drugs of this class?

ANSWERS

1. When an ordinary aspirin tablet is swallowed, the tablet must disintegrate and the aspirin dissolve in the stomach or intestinal fluids before it can be absorbed into the bloodstream. The disintegration and dissolution steps are bypassed by Alka-Seltzer™ because the aspirin is already dissolved in the glass of water before it is consumed. Thus, absorption of aspirin is faster with Alka-Seltzer™ than with ordinary tablets when a single dose of each is consumed. This faster absorption may be useful when an acute effect is desired—such as for a headache.

However, when both products are taken chronically on a regular schedule, the overall bioavailability and steady-state plasma salicylate levels would be expected to be about the same for the two products. After single doses, the plasma level rises more rapidly with Alka-Seltzer™ than with aspirin tablets, but it would also fall off more rapidly. The total area under the curve of plasma level versus time would be about the same for the two products. With repeated doses, the peak to trough variations might be slightly greater with Alka-Seltzer™ than with aspirin, but in general the mean plasma levels would be about the same.

In single doses, Alka-Seltzer™ produces less gastrointestinal bleeding than aspirin tablets, but on a long-term chronic basis this advantage has not been proved. Moreover, there are offsetting disadvantages to Alka-Seltzer™ taken chronically. Alka-Seltzer™ contains citric acid and excess sodium bicarbonate, which react on contact with water to produce the "fizz" of carbon dioxide. The extra sodium (506 mg per tablet) is undesirable on a chronic basis, and so is the tendency to produce systemic alkalosis and an alkaline urine. Also, since Alka-Seltzer must be taken with water, the patient would tend to retain fluid as well as sodium. The alkalinization of the urine will hasten the excretion of aspirin and decrease its therapeutic effect.

Alka-Seltzer™ is much more expensive per unit dose than ordinary aspirin tablets. Generic aspirin tablets (325 mg each) cost about $2.50 for 500 tablets (0.5 cents per tablet), whereas an Alka-Seltzer tablet (aspirin 325 mg, plus sodium bicarbonate 1710 mg, plus citric acid 1220 mg) may cost up to 25 cents each.

2. Because of a saturable step in aspirin's metabolic biotransformation in the liver, an increase in dosage may change the kinetics of plasma disappearance from first order to zero order leading to aspirin accumulation with repeated doses and the development of salicylate toxicity. Some of the signs and symptoms appear to be caused by direct central nervous system effects of aspirin, for example, nausea, vomiting, tinnitus, hyperpnea (increased minute ventilation, with a respiratory alkalosis), and perhaps agitation and confusion. Other signs and symptoms are secondary to the metabolic effects and the acid-base disturbances (metabolic acidosis with an anion gap), for example, paradoxical fever caused by uncoupling of oxidative phosphorylation in the skeletal muscles. The fever increases sweating and cutaneous blood flow (flush). Effects on the circulation may be a result of combined direct (central and peripheral) and indirect actions. The loss of fluids through vomiting, sweating, and breathing may lead to a marked decline in urine output.

We do not have a way to rapidly increase hepatic metabolism. However, total salicylate clearance can be enhanced by maintaining urine output in the normal range (at least 40 ml/hour), and also by making sure that the pH of the urine is in the alkaline range (>7). Salicylic acid will be present in its charged form (salicylate ion) in alkaline urine, will be less likely to be reabsorbed, and thus will be more likely to be eliminated. If the urine is not already alkaline, the patient should be treated with sodium bicarbonate. This will not only hasten the urinary excretion of aspirin and free salicylate, but it will also help clear them from the central nervous system.

3. All NSAID have both analgesic and anti-inflammatory properties, and their approval by the FDA for analgesia, for arthritis therapy, or for both is probably more the result of the manufacturer's marketing strategy than for any rational reasons. The NSAIDs are grouped into seven different classes, based on chemical structure (salicylates plus six other classes). Acetaminophen, which is only weakly anti-inflammatory, is not considered a true anti-inflammatory drug; its analgesic effects are comparable to those of aspirin.

There are no recognizably clear differences among the various NSAIDs. The drugs must be administered from once a day to as often as 5 times per day (based on differences in elimination half-life). Currently, the poorly defined patient-to-patient differences (interpatient variability) may be more significant than drug-to-drug differences. We don't fully understand it, but some patients achieve much more relief with some of these drugs than with others.

SECTION FOUR

DRUGS FOR ENDOCRINE AND METABOLIC DISEASES

CHAPTER 23

DRUGS FOR HYPERURICEMIA AND GOUT

Related Readings

Clark: Chapter 48
Craig and Stitzel: Chapter 71
Gilman et al: Chapter 29, pp. 708-715
Katzung: Chapter 34, pp. 409-413

Key Concepts

- Production of uric acid, mechanism of action of allopurinol
- Renal handling of uric acid, drugs that interfere with renal clearance of uric acid, drug therapy of gout

QUESTIONS

1. A patient is brought into the hospital for treatment of a *lymphoma* (a large tumor of the lymph glands). The drug therapy (chemotherapy) for this type of tumor is very effective, and most of the tumor cells are quickly killed with the first round of chemotherapy. What happens to the cells as they are killed? What steps should be taken to prevent the accumulation of toxic substances?

2. A 65-year-old man sees his doctor for his yearly physical examination. He complains of a few minor joint aches and pains, and is found to have moderate hypertension. His physician recommends that he take aspirin for his joint problems, and prescribes hydrochlorothiazide (a thiazide diuretic) to control his blood pressure. Several weeks later he suddenly develops an intensely painful, red, swollen, hot joint at the base of his large toe. What happened? What is your immediate treatment for this problem? How about long-term management or prevention?

ANSWERS

1. The abrupt death and lysis of perhaps as many as 10^{11} lymphoma cells will suddenly release into the circulation the products resulting from the death of those cells. The most dangerous products released from abruptly dying cells are potassium and DNA degradation products. The DNA, although not toxic itself, is ultimately catabolized to purines and pyrimidines, and the purines are metabolized by xanthine oxidase from hypoxanthine to xanthine to uric acid (Fig. 23-1). The sudden production of large quantities of uric acid can exceed the patient's ability to clear it, and

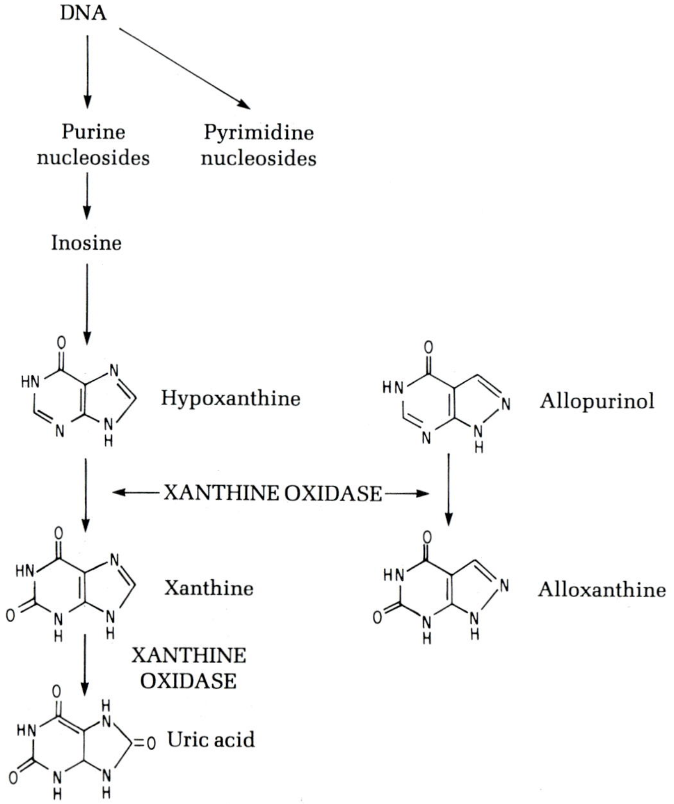

FIG. 23-1. Metabolism of DNA to produce uric acid. Note that inhibition of xanthine oxidase decreases production of the end product, uric acid, and increases excretion of more soluble intermediate products, hypoxanthine and xanthine. Note also that allopurinol is both an inhibitor of xanthine oxidase, and a substrate for the enzyme itself.

severe hyperuricemia may result. Severe hyperuricemia may in turn cause gout, abrupt renal failure, or even death.

Although we cannot prevent the abrupt release of DNA, we can inhibit the production of the toxic end product, uric acid. If the patient is pretreated with allopurinol, an isomer of hypoxanthine and an inhibitor of xanthine oxidase, then the less toxic precursors hypoxanthine and xanthine will be excreted, and less uric acid will be formed (Fig. 23-1). Remember that both hypoxanthine and xanthine are much more soluble in urine than uric acid.

Another approach to protecting the kidneys from acute uric acid nephropathy (sudden damage by precipitation of uric acid) is to maintain a brisk urine flow and to administer enough sodium bicarbonate to maintain an alkaline urine (pH >7.5). Uric acid, being a weak organic acid, is more soluble in alkaline aqueous solutions. Both of these steps will help prevent the excreted uric acid from precipitating in the kidneys and tubules. In fact, all three of these steps (administration of allopurinol, maintenance of good urine output, alkalinization of urine) are used clinically to protect the kidneys.

2. Small to moderate doses of aspirin are known to inhibit the renal tubular secretion of uric acid, and this often leads to a small rise in plasma uric acid levels. The thiazide diuretics are also known to produce hyperuricemia, perhaps secondary to a contraction in extracellular fluid volume. This contraction could lead to increased proximal reabsorption of water and solutes, and increased passive reabsorption of urate. This patient was probably already susceptible to gout and an acute attack was precipitated by the combination of aspirin and hydrochlorothiazide. The drugs should be stopped and treatment for acute gout started.

The drugs of choice for such an acute attack are indomethacin (a NSAID) or colchicine. Most physicians would not start active drug treatment for chronic or recurrent gout unless the patient had a series of several acute attacks. The choices for chronic treatment of either recurrent gout or hyperuricemia would be allopurinol for a patient who overproduces uric acid, or probenecid for a patient who underexcretes uric acid. However, this particular patient would probably not require chronic treatment if the two drugs that precipitated his problem are discontinued.

CHAPTER 24

THYROID REPLACEMENT AND ANTITHYROID DRUGS

Related Readings

Clark et al: Chapter 44
Craig and Stitzel: Chapter 66
Gilman et al: Chapter 60
Katzung: Chapter 37

Key Concepts

- Advantages and disadvantages of different thyroid replacement drugs
- Various therapies to reduce production of T4 by the thyroid gland; use of beta-blockers to relieve symptoms of hyperthyroidism

QUESTIONS

1. A 70-year-old woman with mild angina pectoris had her thyroid gland removed 25 years ago to treat a large goiter. Since then she has taken thyroid tablets USP (65 mg per day) daily to replace her missing endogenous thyroid hormones. She moves to your city and comes to your clinic for ongoing care. You see her in your clinic rotation during your third year, and discover that your hospital's pharmacy does not carry thyroid, USP. You believe she requires continued maintenance, but your pharmacy offers only oral T4 or oral T3 synthetic preparations. Why doesn't your pharmacy stock the "natural" preparation? What would you prescribe for her, and why?

2. A 23-year-old woman develops the most common form of hyperthyroidism—Graves' disease. She complains of fever, sweating, tremor, nervousness, diarrhea, mild weight loss, intolerance of heat, and palpitations. She works as a country and western singer, is married, and has no children. After discussions with her physician, she chooses to be treated with propylthiouracil. Why did she choose this form of therapy over treatment by surgical resection or treatment with radioactive iodine? How does this drug work? How long does it take to work? From your knowledge of pharmacology, could any other drug be given with propylthiouracil (PTU) to help treat her symptoms before the effects of the PTU were evident? What would you tell the young woman to watch out for during the course of treatment with PTU?

ANSWERS

1. It is likely that thyroid tablets will soon lose their USP status, which is accorded to the best established and most widely used drugs for their respective indications. These thyroid tablets are made from defatted, dried and powdered thyroid glands from food animals. At one time they were considered to be a near perfect form of therapy, but today tablets containing synthetic T4 are preferred because they are more stable, they have a constant potency, and they do not cause allergic reactions. These advantages outweigh the slightly higher cost. You should prescribe the synthetic T4 tablets. Since T4 is deiodinated in vivo to yield physiologically appropriate levels of T3, there is no need to supply additional T3. T3 is particularly dangerous in patients with ischemic heart disease. Thus, this case is an excellent example of how a product that is "all natural" is not better!

2. All of this woman's signs and symptoms are classic in cases of hyperthyroidism. She requires some sort of definitive treatment to reduce the gland's production and release of T4 (and T3). Although surgical subtotal thyroid removal is an excellent treatment, she was probably unwilling to accept it because of her career as an entertainer—the surgery could damage the recurrent laryngeal nerve, leading to vocal cord paralysis and the end of her singing career.

The gland could be ablated by giving a dose of radioactive iodine. However, choosing the proper dose is difficult, and persistent hyperthyroidism or hypothyroidism can occur. Also, many young women remain concerned about possible effects of the radioactive iodine upon their future children, even though this concern appears to be only theoretical.

Propylthiouracil (PTU) seems to work by blocking iodine organification and blocking coupling of the iodotyrosines. Since synthesis of new T4, rather than release of previously formed T4, is the affected step, PTU does not appear to "work" for 3 to 4 weeks. One advantage of the treatment with PTU is that it would leave her with an intact gland, and she has a moderate chance of going into a spontaneous remission that would allow her to lead a perfectly normal life. Unfortunately, there is no way to predict in advance which patients will go into remission and which will not. The odds against this outcome may be only 50/50 or even smaller. You should also know that

PTU has certain (uncommon) adverse effects, including rash, vasculitis, or leukopenia.

A drug that is often helpful in controlling *symptoms* of hyperthyroidism is propranolol. It is particularly useful for controlling signs and symptoms that mimic hyperactivity of the sympathetic nervous system on beta-adrenergic receptors (e.g., tachycardia, hypertension, atrial fibrillation). As mentioned above, the most serious side effect of PTU is bone marrow depression with agranulocytosis and intercurrent infection. She should come to see you at the first sign of a sore throat or fever.

CHAPTER 25

INSULIN AND ORAL HYPOGLYCEMIC AGENTS

Related Readings

Clark et al: Chapter 42
Craig and Stitzel: Chapter 68
Gilman et al: Chapter 64
Katzung: Chapter 40

Key Concepts

- Diabetic ketoacidosis: signs and symptoms; management with insulin
- Differences in insulin preparations
- Mode of action, properties of oral hypoglycemic agents

QUESTIONS

1. A 12-year-old child develops a viral illness, and 2 weeks later complains of constant thirst and excessive urination. He then develops nausea, vomiting, dehydration, very heavy breathing, and finally lapses into a coma. When admitted to the hospital, he is noted to be very dehydrated, tachycardic, with deep and rapid respirations. Laboratory studies reveal his blood sugar to be 800 mg/dl (very high) with ketones present in the blood, sugar and ketones present in the urine, and serious metabolic acidosis. What do you think happened to this child? What properties of insulin would be most important to you as you plan to manage his condition?

2. After the boy recovers from this acute illness, you must plan his longterm therapy with insulin. What options do you have in terms of source of insulin? Purity of insulin? Duration of action and time of onset of insulin preparations? Why aren't there just one or two different insulin preparations available?

3. Some patients with diabetes, especially elderly patients who are overweight, have symptoms of diabetes (hyperglycemia, thirst, excessive urination) but have sufficient pancreatic production of insulin that they can avoid the severe acute problems such as hyperglycemic coma or ketoacidosis. What class of drugs can be useful in such patients? How do these drugs work? How can you choose among the half dozen or more drugs of this class?

ANSWERS

1. Perhaps as a result of his viral illness, this child developed type I insulin-dependent (juvenile onset) diabetes mellitus. The virus may have damaged pancreatic beta cells or stimulated an autoimmune reaction against his own beta cells. His condition went unrecognized until he finally went into a severe diabetic crisis with hyperglycemia and ketoacidosis. This child needs immediate treatment with insulin to control both of these problems; fluid and electrolyte replacement will also be necessary. To achieve rapid control and close titration of the blood sugar, you need to find an insulin preparation that can be given intravenously, with rapid onset of action (within minutes) and relatively brief duration of action (minutes to hours). An insulin preparation given subcutaneously, with slow onset and long duration of action, would not provide prompt control.

The best choice of insulin in this situation would be regular (crystalline zinc) insulin injection. This could be given as repeated intravenous injections, repeated subcutaneous injections, or (perhaps optimally) as a continuous intravenous infusion. The source of the insulin (bovine, porcine, mixed, human cloned) and degree of purity (single peak, etc.) would not be critical in this situation, since this patient should not be allergic or resistant to any formulations.

2. Insulin is isolated from the pancreases of cows or pigs, and human insulin has also been synthesized by inserting the genetic coding for human insulin into a cooperative bacterium. The human preparation is more expensive, and is usually not needed unless there are problems with allergy or resistance with one of the animal formulations. There have been recent improvements in purification of insulin from animal sources. Some procedures remove proteins with molecular weights greater than insulin, such as proinsulin, whereas other procedures remove most lower molecular weight contaminants as well. Common formulations have less than 50 ppm proinsulin. If the products have less than 10 ppm, they can be labelled as "purified." Thus, there are at least four sources of insulin available (bovine, porcine, mixed, and human), some of which are available in different degrees of purity.

This situation is made even more confusing because insulin, regardless of source, is prepared in a variety of pharmaceutical formulations that differ in terms of solubility, route of administration, time of onset, and duration of action. Besides the very soluble, rapidly acting, shorter duration preparations described above (useful when rapid changes and close titration are necessary), insulin is available in intermediate and long-acting forms that are less soluble, have slower onsets of action, and more prolonged durations of action. The longer-acting preparations have the advantage of requiring fewer injections throughout the day. Some patients may do well with one or two insulin injections per day, each injection containing a mixture of insulin preparations. Such mixtures may provide for fewer peaks and valleys in blood glucose, and therefore a smoother and more even control of blood glucose.

These varied pharmaceutical preparations of the active agent—insulin—demonstrate how a specific drug or hormone can be formulated in different ways to optimize drug therapy. You will find similar application for pharmaceutical variation when you study the different preparations of penicillin.

3. This type of disease is called Type II, insulin independent or maturity onset diabetes. Although these patients usually do not require insulin therapy, they may respond to weight loss or to the oral hypoglycemic drugs, such as the sulfonylureas. These drugs probably act by stimulating beta cells to release preformed insulin, but they may also reduce glucagon levels or enhance the response of peripheral tissue to circulating levels of insulin by increasing the number of insulin receptors.

Several different oral agents are available, differing in terms of daily dose and half-life of elimination. Chlorpropamide has the longest duration of action, and should probably be avoided in patients with kidney or liver disease. Although a long duration of action is sometimes useful, the toxicity (i.e., hypoglycemia) from an excessive dose can persist for days because of this long half-life of elimination. Some of the newer oral agents are called second generation drugs. They are more potent than the older drugs and seem to have fewer systemic side effects as well. Their exact role in relation to the older drugs is still being determined.

CHAPTER 26

LIPID-LOWERING DRUGS

Related Readings

Clark et al: Chapter 39
Craig and Stitzel: Chapter 23
Gilman et al: Chapter 34
Katzung: Chapter 33

Key Concepts

- Dangers of hypertriglyceridemia, actions of nicotinic acid, side effects of nicotinic acid, difference from nicotinamide
- Dangers of hypercholesterolemia, actions of colestipol, side effects of colestipol

QUESTIONS

1. A 35-year-old man is discovered to have familial hypertriglyceridemia with severe elevation of his triglyceride (TG) levels. Diet alone has not had much effect on lowering his triglyceride levels, so the drug nicotinamide is added. A second physician observes that this is an incorrect drug and changes the prescription. After taking the new drug, the patient develops an uncomfortable sensation of warmth and flushing after each dose. What do you make of this story?

2. A 40-year-old man is found to have high levels of cholesterol with associated tendinous xanthomatosis and xanthelasma. These problems were noted when he suffered his first myocardial infarction at a relatively early age. Since his cholesterol level was 450 mg/dl, it was assumed that he had inherited the heterozygous form of familial hypercholesterolemia. Dietary education was given, and treatment with colestipol was begun. How does this drug work in this condition? Should the drug be discontinued when constipation develops?

ANSWERS

1. The first physician confused nicotinamide with nicotinic acid. They are equally potent as vitamins, but only the latter drug lowers blood lipids. Nicotinic acid probably works by inhibiting very low–density lipoprotein (VLDL) secretion, in turn decreasing the production of low–density lipoprotein (LDL), and thereby decreasing serum levels of triglycerides. The drug has no effect on production of bile acids, and does little to lower serum cholesterol levels.

The warm flush is a characteristic side effect of nicotinic acid when it is taken in the megadoses required to lower blood lipids. This effect appears to be mediated by an effect of nicotinic acid on prostaglandin synthesis in cutaneous blood vessels. Interestingly, this effect can be prevented by taking aspirin. In addition, continued use of the drug usually leads to a reduction (tachyphylaxis) of this side effect.

This case demonstrates the importance of ordering a drug in the correct form. The chemical difference between nicotinic acid and nicotinamide is small (Fig. 26-1), but it is important to this patient.

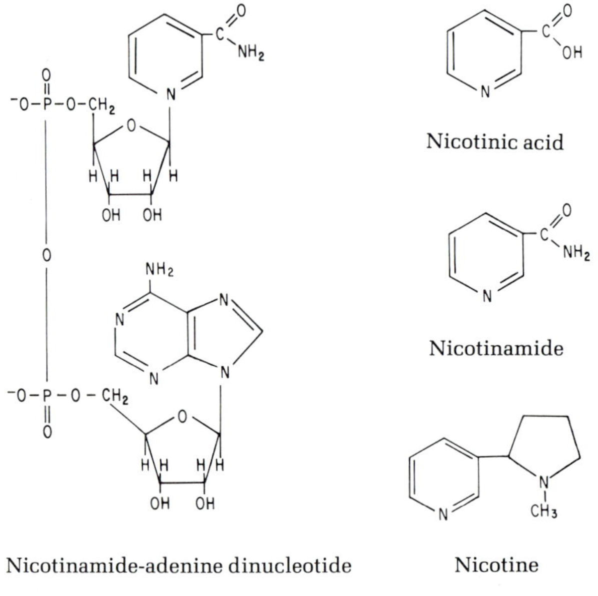

FIG. 26-1. Structures of nicotinic acid and nicotinamide. Both drugs are effective forms of the vitamin, since both can be converted to nicotinamide adenine dinucleotide (NAD), also pictured. However, only nicotinic acid (also called niacin) in high doses has a lipid-lowering effect. Incidentally, niacin was a term introduced to avoid confusion with a totally unrelated alkaloid, nicotine, also shown.

2. Patients with moderately severe hypercholesterolemia are at risk for developing cholesterol deposits along tendons and around the eyes, and for developing early onset coronary artery disease. Hypercholesterolemia is an independent and important risk factor for coronary artery disease, along with more widely known risk factors, such as smoking and hypertension.

Colestipol is a bile-sequestering agent used to reduce serum cholesterol levels. As an anion exchange resin, it is insoluble in water and not absorbed systemically. It exchanges chloride ions for anionic bile acids in the intestine, preventing reabsorption of the latter. Since bile acids inhibit cholesterol catabolism, this "brake" mechanism is released and cholesterol is broken down more rapidly into bile acids leading to a decreased serum level of cholesterol.

Many such resins, which are not absorbed, tend to cause constipation. If constipation develops in the absence of frank intestinal obstruction, you may want to add a laxative to the colestipol, but in most cases you should be able to continue this treatment. Indeed, this treatment may be very important in helping to prevent further atherosclerosis and a second myocardial infarction.

CHAPTER 27

VITAMINS

Related Readings

Clark et al: Chapter 50
Craig and Stitzel: Chapter 75
Gilman et al: Chapters 66 and 67
Katzung: Chapter 21, pp. 256-257; Chapter 65, pp. 772-773

Key Concepts

- Role of thiamine, symptoms of thiamine deficiency
- Role of retinol, symptoms of retinol excess

QUESTIONS

1. A 60-year-old alcoholic man was brought to the VA hospital by his landlady. She had observed that he consumed large quantities of beer, often in excess of 12 cans per day. His diet consisted largely of peanuts, pretzels, potato chips, and other junk food. She noticed that he had complained of muscular pain, weakness, and funny feelings in his hands and feet. His ankles had begun to be puffy with fluid, and he had recently shown jerky movements of his eyes, and had been bumping into furniture. Most recently, he had become totally incapable of remembering anything at all, and he seemed to make up stories to answer questions. What would you prescribe for this patient in addition to abstinence from alcohol?

2. A 35-year-old woman was admitted to the hospital for the diagnosis and treatment of a gradual onset of anorexia, nausea, vomiting, and severe diffuse headache. She had also noted dry, itching, and red skin, and some hair loss. She was taking no prescription medications or recreational drugs. Her physical examination revealed mild papilledema (swelling of the optic discs), suggesting the presence of increased intracranial pressure. This finding, together with her history, strongly suggested the presence of a brain tumor, but a CT scan of the head was negative. At this point, the medical student discovered in a more detailed history that she was taking a medication, but since it was available without a prescription, she had forgotten to mention it and no one had specifically asked. What do you think she was taking?

ANSWERS

1. Alcoholics who drink only their alcoholic beverage(s) with little consumption of normal foods are at risk for several vitamin deficiency syndromes that can be life threatening. Not only is dietary intake affected, but malabsorption of some of the water-soluble vitamins can also occur.

The symptoms in this case suggest a diagnosis of thiamine deficiency, which is common in alcoholics. Thiamine is most plentiful in foods such as meats, wheat germ, grains, cereals, and bread—you can see why a deficiency might occur. The active form of thiamine is thiamine pyrophosphate, which is important in carbohydrate metabolism.

Thiamine deficiency can present in a number of different ways. Polyneuritis is often seen in patients with a mild deficiency, whereas beriberi heart disease (high cardiac output, vasodilatation, edema) may occur in more severe cases. Wernicke's encephalopathy is a severe neurologic problem that includes ophthalmoplegia (inability to move the eyes fully), nystagmus (jerky, rhythmic movements of the eyes), ataxia (clumsiness), global mental deterioration, and even coma. Korsakoff's syndrome consists of retrograde amnesia, poor ability to learn, confabulation, and even a frank psychosis. When these two neurologic syndromes blend with one another, it is referred to as the Wernicke-Korsakoff syndrome. This syndrome represents a medical emergency that must be promptly recognized and treated with thiamine (100 mg intravenously).

2. Excessive intake of retinol (vitamin A) can cause a syndrome closely mimicking the presentation of a brain tumor, with headache, loss of appetite, nausea, vomiting, increased intracranial pressure, and even neurologic signs. However, CT scans of the brain are negative. Retinol excess can also cause the skin and hair problems described.

This woman read in a health magazine that vitamin A might help prevent cancer (an interesting but currently unproven hypothesis). At her supermarket or health food store she purchased tablets that contained four times the recommended daily allowance of the vitamin, and took 4 or 5 of these tablets every day for several months. As she gradually developed vitamin A excess, she began to develop the symptoms of hypervitaminosis A.

Vitamin A performs many essential functions in the body (effects on vision, skin, mucous membranes, and bones), but vitamin A deficiency is extremely uncommon in the United States (it is a problem in many other areas of the world, however). Over the last few years, massive ingestion of pure vitamin preparations by health food or vitamin enthusiasts has led to the recognition that some hypervitaminosis states are quite serious. Since these vitamin preparations are available without prescription, and "megavitamin therapy" seems to be more popular, we will likely see more such cases in the future.

SECTION FIVE

ANESTHETIC AGENTS

CHAPTER 28

GENERAL ANESTHESIA I

Related Readings

Clark et al: Chapter 32
Craig and Stitzel: Chapters 30 and 31
Gilman et al: Chapters 13 and 14
Katzung: Chapter 23

Key Concepts

- Lability of inhalational anesthetics
- Differences in anesthetic properties among ethyl ether, nitrous oxide, and halothane

QUESTIONS

1. If you were designing an optimal inhalational anesthetic agent, you would want it to cause rapid induction and allow rapid emergence from the anesthetized state (so called lability or maneuverability). Which three properties of an inhalational agent contribute to its ability to "start and stop" quickly? Conversely, which three properties of an inhalational agent make it slow to turn on and off? Discuss these properties as they apply to diethyl ether, nitrous oxide, and halothane.

2. The following three classic inhalational anesthetic agents have been used over the years: ethyl ether, nitrous oxide, and halothane. As head of the formulary committee for your small hospital, you must choose to stock only one of these agents. What six criteria would you use to select the "best" agent? Make a 3 × 6 table to summarize how these six criteria apply to these three agents.

ANSWERS

1. The greatest lability (maneuverability) of a gaseous general anesthetic is provided by a combination of: (1) high potency or a low partial gas pressure in the lungs (alveoli) for effective induction and maintenance of anesthesia (low minimum alveolar anesthetic concentration, or MAC); (2) a low degree of solubility in fluid (blood) so that the blood capacity for the agent is relatively small (low blood:gas partition coefficient); and (3) a low degree of solubility in the brain and in lipids, so that the capacity of these compartments for the gas is relatively small (low brain:blood partition coefficient). The opposite properties, namely low potency, high fluid solubility, and high fat solubility, result in agents that require long periods for induction and emergence from anesthesia.

Anesthesiologists prefer to use inhalational agents with prompt induction and emergence properties, and patients are also more likely to prefer agents that result in prompt induction. The values of these important properties for the three classic general anesthetic agents are given below:

Agent	MAC %	Blood:gas partition coefficient	Brain:blood partition coefficient
Diethyl ether	10	>10	1.1
Nitrous oxide	105	0.47	1.1
Halothane	0.75	2.30	2.9

As you can see, induction and emergence from general anesthesia would be faster with nitrous oxide than with halothane (lower partition coefficients). However, nitrous oxide cannot be used by itself to provide general anesthesia, since its MAC is greater than 100% (at standard atmospheric pressure).

2. The six properties that are often used to compare inhalational agents include the following: (1) effectiveness (achievable depth of anesthesia); (2) reversibility (lability of anesthesia, as discussed in the question above); (3) potency (the partial pressure of the gas required to provide general anesthesia, or MAC); (4) toxicity (acute and chronic effects of administration); (5) flammability (explosion hazard posed by the gas or vapor); and (6) acceptability (as reported by the patient, in terms of odor, taste, membrane irritation, bad dreams). Those six criteria are applied to the three classic agents in the following list:

Properties	**Ether**	**N_2O**	**Halothane**
Effectiveness	Good	Poor	Good
Reversibility	Slow	Most rapid	Rapid
Potency (MAC)	10%	105%	1%
Toxicity	Low	Low	Moderate
Flammability	Yes	No	No
Acceptability	Low	Good	Good

Most hospitals have several inhalational agents available in the operating room, since different procedures and different patients require a variety of approaches to anesthesia. However, this type of analysis demonstrates why ether is used so rarely today, even though it remains highly effective as a single agent.

CHAPTER 29

GENERAL ANESTHESIA II

Related Readings

Clark et al: Chapter 32
Craig and Stitzel: Chapters 30 and 31
Gilman et al: Chapters 13 and 14
Katzung: Chapter 23

Key Concepts

- Anesthetic properties of nitrous oxide, use of induction agents, use of paralyzing agents, use of balanced anesthesia
- Use of anticholinergic agents, histamine antagonists, sedatives, and antibiotics in conjunction with general anesthesia

QUESTIONS

1. As you are reviewing the anesthesia record of a patient in the hospital, you note that the principal anesthetic agent used was nitrous oxide. Several other drugs were used as well: thiopental given intravenously during induction, inhaled oxygen, and fentanyl, droperidol, and tubocurarine given intravenously. Why were all these other agents necessary? Why not use just nitrous oxide?

2. Before he is taken to the operating room to have a fractured hip nailed, your uncle receives the following intravenous medications: glycopyrrolate, cimetidine, lorazepam, and cefazolin. What kinds of drugs are these, and why are they being given "on call" to the operating room?

ANSWERS

1. Nitrous oxide has excellent lability for an inhalational agent, but induction with intravenous thiopental is even more rapid. Loss of consciousness after intravenous administration of thiopental usually occurs in just a few seconds. This type of very quick induction is preferred by most patients.

Because nitrous oxide has such a low potency (MAC = 105%), it cannot be used (without a hyperbaric chamber) by itself to provide total anesthesia. The patient may develop hypoxemia unless supplemental oxygen is given during the procedure. During emergence diffusion hypoxia may result, so it is common to give the patient 100% oxygen to breathe.

Fentanyl is an opioid analgesic that decreases the tendency for pain to lessen the level of anesthesia during the procedure, and to help relieve immediate postoperative pain. When opioids or sedative-hypnotics are used in conjunction with an inhalational agent such as nitrous oxide, this is called "balanced" anesthesia, and it helps compensate for the inability of nitrous oxide to provide complete anesthesia when used alone.

Droperidol is a neuroleptic (antipsychotic) drug that may be useful during general anesthesia for its ability to provide an element of "dissociative" anesthesia and for its antiemetic effects. Vomiting is dangerous during anesthesia because of the risk of aspiration.

Finally, tubocurarine was given to promote muscle relaxation, which would make the surgery easier.

As you can see, an ideal inhalational agent could be given alone and provide satisfactory performance in all the above areas. In the case of nitrous oxide, help in the form of other drugs is needed to provide a satisfactory course of inhalational anesthesia. This is an example of the deliberate use of drug interactions to help the patient experience drug effects that would not be achievable by the use of nitrous oxide as a single general anesthetic agent.

2. Glycopyrrolate is a synthetic anticholinergic (muscarinic receptor blocking drug) that is also a quaternary ammonium compound. Because it is always charged, it does not penetrate the blood-brain barrier and it lacks the central nervous system effects of atropine or scopolamine. It was given to prevent excess salivary flow and it also reduces airway secretions, although this is not usually a problem with nitrous oxide. It would block excessive secretion of gastric acid, which also results from excessive vagal activity. At the same time, it seems to cause less tachycardia than atropine.

Cimetidine is an H_2 (histamine) receptor blocking drug that would also prevent excessive secretion of gastric acid secondary to vagal activity during the procedure. By raising the pH of gastric secretions before surgery, any accidental aspiration of gastric fluids would produce less severe aspiration pneumonitis.

Lorazepam is a sedative-hypnotic drug of the benzodiazepine class. Its anti-anxiety effects would help calm the patient; its sedative-hypnotic effects would add to that of the nitrous oxide, which has such a low potency that it often needs to be supplemented with other agents; and its muscle relaxant effects may add to that of the curare.

Finally, cefazolin is a so-called "first-generation" cephalosporin antibiotic. In some types of surgery where the risk of a postoperative wound infection is high, or where a prosthetic device is inserted (such as the metal nail in the hip), its administration before surgery lowers the chance of postoperative wound infection. You can see again that the whole process of anesthesia is a complicated one in which many deliberate drug interactions occur, and intimate knowledge of the pharmacology of these agents is necessary to choose the safest and best combination of drugs.

CHAPTER 30

LOCAL ANESTHETICS

Related Readings

Clark et al: Chapter 33
Craig and Stitzel: Chapter 33
Gilman et al: Chapter 15
Katzung: Chapter 24

Key Concepts

- Amide and ester classes of local anesthetics
- Central nervous system effects of local anesthetics

QUESTIONS

1. You may have a childhood memory of going to the dentist and receiving a shot of a drug called Novocain™. This is a local anesthetic of the "ester" class. What is the generic name for Novocain™? What other local anesthetics are in this class? After you draw the structure of Novocain™, discuss its metabolic fate. Why are drugs of this class used less often than drugs of the "amide" class?

2. A medical student decided to have his two impacted wisdom teeth extracted on an outpatient basis. Local anesthesia was accomplished with several injections (local infiltrations, nerve blocks) of lidocaine hydrochloride 2% solution. However, the initial blocks were not entirely satisfactory and two more injections were required, for a total volume of 15 ml. After the fourth injection, the student began to complain of lightheadedness, visual problems, and restlessness. He then suddenly developed tonic-clonic seizures while in the chair. How much lidocaine did he receive? How do you explain these symptoms and signs? How should they be treated? Is there any way to slow the absorption of lidocaine or to prevent seizures if large doses must be given?

ANSWERS

1. The United States Adopted Name (USAN) for Novocain™ is procaine. However, some dentists may say Novocain™ when they mean any type of local anesthetic, not necessarily procaine. Other ester-type local anesthetics include chloroprocaine and tetracaine. Cocaine is also in this class, although it is no longer used therapeutically as a local anesthetic. The structure of these local anesthetics is seen in Fig. 30-1.

The ester bond of procaine is hydrolyzed by serum cholinesterase to yield para-aminobenzoic acid (PABA) and diethylaminoethanol. The ester

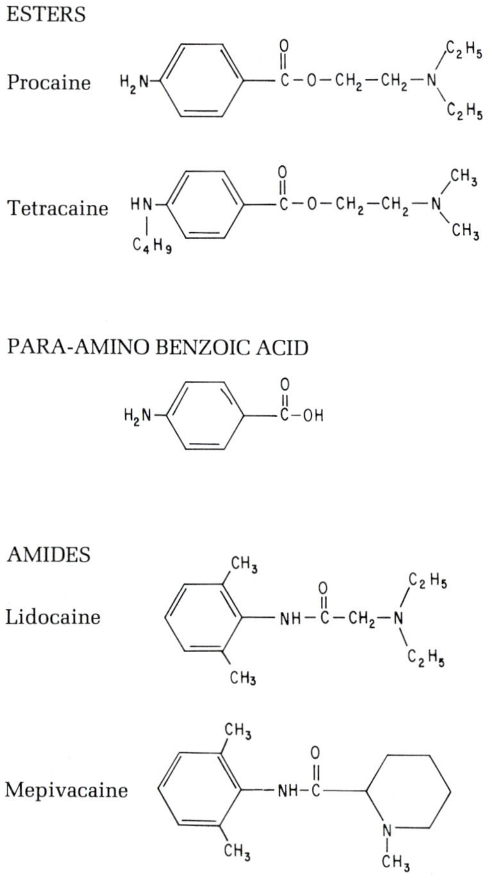

FIG. 30-1. The chemical structures of several local anesthetics. Note the difference between the amide agents and the ester agents. Also, note the structure of the metabolite of the ester-class agents, para-aminobenzoic acid (PABA).

type local anesthetics are more likely to produce hypersensitivity reactions (allergic dermatitis, asthma, anaphylaxis) because most of these reactions are due to the metabolite, PABA. The amide-type local anesthetics such as lidocaine are not split by plasma cholinesterase, and are not metabolized to PABA (see Fig. 30-1). Thus, they are more commonly used because of their longer duration of action, and decreased incidence of acute allergic reactions.

2. A 2% solution of lidocaine hydrochloride contains 2 g/100 ml, which equals 2,000 mg/100 ml or 20 mg/ml. The student received a total of 15 ml, which is equivalent to 300 mg of the drug. This dose is comparable to the usual intravenous dose of 100 to 200 mg given to control ventricular arrhythmias. Remember that the tissues in the mouth, especially the tongue, are very vascular and lidocaine may be rapidly absorbed through the extensive venous system. The signs and symptoms are typical of lidocaine toxicity, and they are caused by direct central nervous system (CNS) effects (CNS stimulation because of suppression of inhibitory neurons). The patient should be treated with a rapidly acting CNS depressant drug that has anticonvulsant activity. A good choice would be intravenous diazepam.

The dose of lidocaine can be kept restricted to the area where local anesthesia is desired by incorporating a vasoconstrictor into the lidocaine solution. This will reduce blood flow to the area and reduce the rate of absorption of lidocaine. Epinephrine is often used for this purpose. Occasionally, when large doses of lidocaine are needed, the patient can also be sedated with diazepam, which has the added advantage of helping to suppress potential seizures.

This "trick" of slowing lidocaine absorption by adding epinephrine is useful, but it must not be used in areas of the body where the resultant vasoconstriction could cause serious problems. For example, lidocaine with epinephrine must never be used in tissues such as the fingers, toes, ears, or nose.

SECTION SIX

DRUGS ACTING ON THE CENTRAL NERVOUS SYSTEM

CHAPTER 31

OPIOID ANALGESICS I

Related Readings

Clark et al: Chapter 29
Craig and Stitzel: Chapter 43
Gilman et al: Chapter 22
Katzung: Chapter 29

Key Concepts

- Difference between the terms "narcotic" and "opioid"
- Differences among opioid agonists, partial agonists, and pure antagonists

QUESTIONS

1. Why is the term *opioid analgesic* preferable to the term *narcotic analgesic?*

2. You are interviewing a patient who has had extensive recreational experience with opioid agents. He tells you that morphine gives him a "rush;" codeine gives him less of a rush; nalbuphine gives even less of a rush, and if he takes it before morphine, actually reduces the pleasure associated with morphine; and taking naloxone gives no pleasure at all, but does block the rush of morphine if he takes naloxone before he takes the morphine. How do you explain this patient's observations?

ANSWERS

1. A narcotic is an agent that produces narcosis or a stuporous state, whereas the opiates, which are derived from opium or are chemically modified, produce analgesia without the deliberate loss of consciousness. Opioids refer to all such analgesic agents whether natural or synthetic. Many agents relieve pain because they produce unconsciousness (e.g., halothane, thiopental), but they lack the pharmacologic specificity of the opioids. When we use opioids, we usually wish to provide analgesia without causing sleepiness (e.g., for a patient who is working and has a painful broken ankle), and thus we should not refer to these drugs as narcotics. When opiods produce drowsiness, this is a side effect, not usually the desired therapeutic effect.

2. It is still not clear which particular type of opioid receptor in the human central nervous system is associated with the euphoric effects of morphine-like agonists, although some evidence suggests that mu receptors may be predominantly responsible. Codeine (Fig. 31-1) has a lower affinity

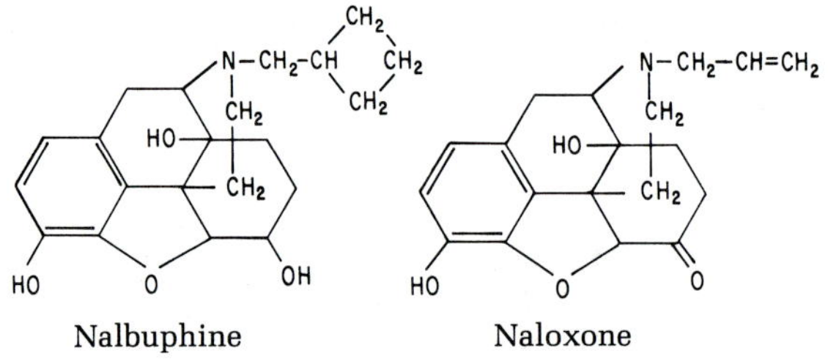

FIG. 31-1. The structures of several opioids. Note the similarity of structure between morphine (strong agonist), codeine (weak agonist), nalbuphine (partial agonist), and naloxone (pure antagonist).

for opioid receptors, and it is probably less effective in activating the receptors associated with euphoria. It may also stimulate other receptors associated with dysphoria and nausea. However, other factors such as lipid solubility, distribution, and metabolism may also play a role. Note that the structural difference between codeine and morphine is simply the replacement of a hydroxy group by a methoxy group.

Nalbuphine is an opioid partial agonist, which means that it has both agonist and antagonist (blocking) actions. It is an effective agonist like morphine, but its euphoric and respiratory depressant effects seem to demonstrate a "ceiling" effect, making it less likely to cause severe respiratory depression. However, these antagonist effects allow it to block the euphoric effects of morphine, and even precipitate a withdrawal reaction in an addict. Again, note how structurally similar nalbuphine is to morphine.

Finally, naloxone is a pure antagonist, and therefore it has no analgesic or sedating effects of its own. However, it can competitively block all the actions of morphine. Opioid antagonists can be used beneficially to counter the effects of an opioid overdose.

CHAPTER 32

OPIOID ANALGESICS II

Related Readings

Clark et al: Chapters 29 and 30, pp. 337-342
Craig and Stitzel: Chapters 43 and 44, pp. 610-616
Gilman et al: Chapters 22 and 23, pp. 532-545
Katzung: Chapters 29 and 30, pp. 350-352

Key Concepts

- Morphine as a drug of abuse, Controlled Substances Act, scheduled substances
- Endogenous opioids

QUESTIONS

1. For any chemical liable to be abused, the physician must be especially aware of the following six properties: (1) acute intoxication, (2) development of tolerance, (3) development of dependence, (4) withdrawal reactions, (5) ability to produce addiction, and (6) medical and social complications of abuse. Consider the abuse of morphine with respect to these six areas. Should morphine be included in the drugs covered by the Controlled Substances Act? If so, under what schedule?

2. Endocrinologists claim that the discipline of pharmacology is actually contained within the field of endocrinology. They argue that all drugs work by way of specific receptors. The receptors must be there to be stimulated by endogenous substances called hormones. Recently exogenous substances (drugs) have been discovered that could stimulate these natural receptors. For example, glucocorticoid receptors are naturally stimulated by hydrocortisone (cortisol), but we have recently designed synthetic drugs such as dexamethasone that are even more potent. If the endocrinologists are correct, what is the evidence that endogenous morphine-like substances exist? Do these substances produce any medically important effects?

ANSWERS

1. The major hazard arising from acute intoxication with opioid analgesics is central respiratory depression, which can progress to the point of complete respiratory arrest. Other effects apparent during acute intoxication include a "rush," sedation ("nod"), apathy, small pupils, and decreased bowel sounds.

The development of tolerance to the euphoric effects leads the drug user to increase the dosage, and the tolerance to respiratory depression allows the user to do that and not show signs of overdose. This is the most important effect to which addicts become tolerant, and it accounts for their ability to survive a dose that would be lethal in a nontolerant human. Other effects of morphine to which humans become tolerant are analgesia and euphoria, but no tolerance develops to the pupilloconstrictive effects or the itching sensation.

Eventually physical and psychologic dependence develop. Psychologic dependence implies that the patient "craves" the drug, whereas physical dependence implies that if the drug is abruptly discontinued, a withdrawal reaction will occur. The addict may now be using the drug as much to prevent the unpleasant syndrome of withdrawal as for its euphoric effects. The withdrawal reaction in opioid analgesic addiction is unpleasant but not usually life-threatening, in contrast to alcohol or barbiturate withdrawal. The withdrawal reaction ("cold turkey") includes malaise, nausea, vomiting, abdominal pain, moist skin with piloerection ("goose bumps"), dilated pupils, nasal congestion, and other symptoms as well.

Addiction is not a precise medical term, but it usually implies that the addict's life is taken over or consumed by the desire to obtain and self-administer the drug. Addiction can occur with or without the development of tolerance or physical dependence. If the morphine addict was regularly provided with a pure and standard potency preparation, he would be able to function almost normally in society. This is one of the reasons for the success of methadone substitution programs, although methadone has other advantages for that purpose.

Most of the medical complications of addiction result from impure drug material (foreign body reactions), unknown potency (risk of respiratory depression and death), and infection (hepatitis, AIDS, endocarditis). The social complications of morphine or heroin abuse result from the high cost of maintaining a constant supply of the drug, which almost always necessitates criminal activity.

Morphine has a very high abuse potential when taken recreationally, but not when given therapeutically to patients in the hospital. Because of this potential for abuse, morphine is covered by the Controlled Substances Act, and all who prescribe or dispense the drug must have a special license from the Drug Enforcement Administration. The drugs with legitimate medical uses that are most likely to be abused are included in Schedule II (opioids, amphetamines, barbiturates); drugs in Schedules III, IV, and V are less likely to be abused.

2. The endocrinologist's argument that drugs work through receptors is probably true for most drugs, but we know less about some receptors than others. Three distinct families of endogenous opioid peptides have been identified: the enkephalins, the endorphins, and the dynorphins. Their distributions, not only in the brain but in other parts of the body as well, follow the patterns of distribution of opioid receptors. They mimic the effects of morphine on those receptors *in vivo* and in isolated systems. They can be shown to bind competitively to those receptors with respect to both agonists and antagonists. Physiologically they appear to function as neurotransmitters, modulators of neurotransmission or neurohormones, but their role is still not well understood. Although this field is still evolving, it has been proposed that the runner's "high" and pain relief from placebos may be caused by the effects of endogenous endorphins on opioid receptors.

CHAPTER 33

CENTRAL NERVOUS SYSTEM PEPTIDES

Related Readings

Clark et al: Chapter 46
Craig and Stitzel: Chapter 62, pp. 866-868
Gilman et al: Chapter 37
Katzung: Chapter 36, pp. 433-435

Key Concepts

- Actions of vasopressin
- Properties of oxytocin

QUESTIONS

1. During your medical rotation through the VA hospital, you assume the care of a 55-year-old male alcoholic who has severe liver cirrhosis. As a complication, he has portal venous hypertension, which has led to dilatation of veins in the esophagus (esophageal varices). One of these veins ruptures and the patient starts to vomit blood; you are told to try to reduce the rate of blood loss by giving intravenous vasopressin. What is this peptide? How does it work in this situation? Why does the patient's mean arterial pressure not increase? Would you see any effect on free water clearance? If the patient had angina, would that be affected?

2. A patient was receiving an intravenous infusion of Pitressin™ at a rate of 0.4 units/minute to control his bleeding from esophageal varices. Because the intensive care unit was full, the patient was sent to the floor while on this drip. A new bottle of the infusate was prepared by a nurse unfamiliar with the preparation, and the new infusate was administered at the same rate of 0.4 units/minute. Shortly after the infusion of the new bottle was started, the patient experienced cardiopulmonary arrest. The first doctor on the scene observed that the new infusate had been prepared from a vial of Pitocin™. What do you think happened?

ANSWERS

1. Vasopressin is another name for antidiuretic hormone (ADH), which is normally released by the posterior pituitary gland in response to hyperosmolality or hypotension. This nonapeptide hormone possesses both antidiuretic and vasopressor properties, as the two names suggest. It is the drug of choice for pituitary diabetes insipidus, but it has another interesting indication. The use of synthetic vasopressin to control hemorrhage caused by ruptured esophageal varices is somewhat controversial, but it is often used because of its ability to constrict splanchnic vessels and reduce portal blood flow. This is a nice example of using a drug for one indication when the drug was initially designed to be used for an entirely different medical problem. Interestingly, vasopressin also has the unexpected effect of facilitating blood clotting.

Vasopressin has only moderate effects on systemic resistance vessels in usual doses, so that it is not as effective in raising the blood pressure as an alpha-adrenergic receptor agonist. In addition, if the pressure began to increase, there might well be a reflex slowing of the heart rate, which would lower the blood pressure again. The antidiuretic effect of vasopressin would be expected to decrease free water clearance. Vasopressin also has semi-selective vasoconstrictor effects in the coronary arteries, so that angina could worsen or develop in patients with coronary artery disease. Remember that even though you may think of vasopressin as a "central nervous system peptide," it is often administered for its systemic effects and its toxic effects usually occur in organs outside the central nervous system.

2. This is a bizarre story that occurred because of a sequence of errors. The patient should have been receiving vasopressin, which has the trade name Pitressin™. Oxytocin has a similar sounding trade name, Pitocin™, but it is a nonapeptide hormone from the posterior pituitary that elicits milk ejection in lactating women. In pharmacologic doses, it is used to induce or accelerate uterine contractions and to help control postpartum hemorrhage. When used in this way, it is administered intravenously in doses of 5 to 20 mUnits/minute.

The pharmacist mistakenly sent Pitocin™ rather than Pitressin™ to the floor. The nurse was not familiar with either drug, and so prepared the infusate with Pitocin™ and began to infuse it at the ordered rate of 0.4 units/

minute (equal to 400 mUnits/minute). This represented a massive overdose (40 times the usual dosage) of oxytocin, which was not the correct drug in any event. Although the exact type of cardiopulmonary arrest was not recorded, it presumably was a consequence of this massive overdose of oxytocin.

Unfortunately, it is not enough to understand the actions of each drug. In addition, you must be constantly on the lookout for accidental confusion between two drugs that have similar names. This episode led the hospital pharmacy to not only store these drugs by generic name rather than trade name, but to store them in physically separate areas to minimize the risk of confusion in the future.

CHAPTER 34

CENTRAL NERVOUS SYSTEM NEUROTRANSMISSION

Related Readings

Clark et al: Chapter 23
Craig and Stitzel: Chapter 29
Gilman et al: Chapter 12
Katzung: Chapter 19

Key Concepts

- Properties of a central nervous system neurotransmitter
- Specific properties of known nonpeptide neurotransmitters
- Handling of neurotransmitters at the synapse

QUESTIONS

1. You are reviewing a scientific paper in which the author claims to have discovered a new endogenous chemical that acts as a neurotransmitter within the central nervous system. What criteria would you look for within the report to convince you that the claim was true?

2. What nonpeptide substances are now fairly well established as being physiologically important central nervous system neurotransmitters? What properties do these transmitters share in common? What three important diseases seem to be associated with (perhaps caused by) deficiencies of these neurotransmitters?

3. Many drugs that act on the central, peripheral, or autonomic nervous systems have their predominant effects near the synapse. Such drugs may act on the presynaptic neuron, on the post-synaptic cell, or in the synapse itself. What are the possible sites at which drugs can alter synaptic transmission, and give an example of a clinically important drug that acts at each site.

ANSWERS

1. To prove that an endogenous chemical is in fact a central nervous system neurotransmitter it would have to be shown that: (1) the chemical was actually present in central nervous system neurons; (2) the enzymes necessary for its synthesis and intermediates in the biosynthetic pathway were present in neurons; (3) mechanisms exist for its rapid catabolism or termination of its action (e.g., re-uptake); (4) the chemical is released when the neuron is stimulated; (5) the exogenous chemical applied postsynaptically mimics the effects of nerve stimulation; and (6) other related agonists and antagonists can be found or synthesized. Overall, not a simple task!

2. Nonpeptide substrates with well-established roles as central nervous system transmitters include dopamine, norepinephrine, epinephrine, serotonin, acetylcholine, γ-aminobutyric acid (GABA), and glycine. All of these meet the criteria above.

Parkinsonism appears to be caused by a specific deficiency of dopamine-producing neurons that form synapses in the basal ganglia. Psychiatric depression seems to be associated with a deficit in noradrenergic transmission in the brain. One theory about the pathogenesis of Alzheimer's disease suggests that it is associated with a deficit in cholinergic transmission.

3. The sites and mechanisms by which drugs can alter synaptic transmission include the following: (1) drugs may alter the action potential of the presynaptic fiber (e.g., local anesthetics decrease transmission along sensory fibers entering the brainstem and spinal cord); (2) drugs may inhibit the synthesis of transmitter (e.g., synthesis of norepinephrine is inhibited by alpha-methyl-para-tyrosine); (3) drugs may decrease the storage of transmitter (e.g., storage of norepinephrine in adrenergic nerve terminals is decreased by reserpine); (4) drugs may inhibit the catabolism of a transmitter inside the neuron (e.g., monoamine oxidase inhibitors block the catabolism of catecholamines); (5) drugs may block the release of a transmitter (e.g., bretylium blocks the release of norepinephrine); (6) drugs may block the re-uptake of a transmitter (e.g., cocaine blocks the re-uptake of norepinephrine); (7) drugs may inhibit the catabolism of a transmitter in the synapse (e.g., cholinesterase inhibitors such as physostigmine block the breakdown of acetylcholine in the synapse); (8) drugs can block postsynaptic receptors (e.g., propranolol blocks beta-adrenergic receptors); and (9) drugs may block ion channels in postsynaptic receptors that are coupled to excitatory neurotransmitters (e.g., diazepam appears to have this property at GABAergic synapses).

Thus, many important drugs achieve their pharmacologic properties by acting either presynaptically, in the synapse, or postsynaptically.

CHAPTER 35

BENZODIAZEPINES

Related Readings

Clark et al: Chapter 26, pp. 280-286
Craig and Stitzel: Chapter 35, pp. 500-504
Gilman et al: Chapter 17, pp. 339-351
Katzung: Chapter 20

Key Concepts

- Hypnotic properties of different benzodiazepines
- Different metabolic pathways and drug interactions of benzodiazepines
- Metabolism, half-life, and accumulation of benzodiazepines

QUESTIONS

1. Would triazolam, temazepam, or diazepam be the hypnotic of choice for patients with insomnia? How did you make your decision?

2. Two women prone to panic attacks are maintained chronically on benzodiazepines, one on lorazepam and the other on diazepam. Both show good improvement and little central nervous system depression. Both women are started on oral cimetidine to treat suspected ulcers. What do you think will happen?

3. A 79-year-old alcoholic man suffering from acute ethanol withdrawal is admitted to the VA hospital. He is treated with diazepam 5 mg by mouth 4 times daily. This doesn't "hold" him, so his dosage is increased to 10 mg by mouth 4 times daily. By the third day, he starts to calm down and is well enough to be discharged on the fourth day. His discharge medications include diazepam 10 mg 4 times daily and multivitamins once per day.

One week after discharge, his landlady finds him stuporous in his bed, barely responsive to shouted commands. He is brought to your emergency room, and a brief initial evaluation (including what?) fails to determine the cause of his coma. Any ideas?

ANSWERS

1. Both triazolam and temazepam are commonly used for hypnosis (to help induce sleep). Diazepam has a long elimination half-life (1 to 4 days) and two active metabolites. It should be avoided because of the possibility of its accumulation with repeated dosing which would contribute to drug hangover and daytime somnolence.

Triazolam has the shortest elimination half-life of the three (3 to 5 hours), and thus is the least likely to contribute to daytime somnolence the next day. It has the advantage that it is rapidly absorbed after oral ingestion, and thus would work quickly. Its disadvantages are that the sleep may not be of sufficient duration (early waking), and if physical dependence develops, the shorter acting drugs are associated with more intense withdrawal signs.

Temazepam has an intermediate half-life of elimination (5 to 8 hours), which would seem to be ideal for this indication. One of its disadvantages is that it is more slowly absorbed after oral ingestion than triazolam, and thus its hypnotic effect may take longer to develop. It is clear that each of these drugs has relative advantages and disadvantages, based on pharmacokinetic properties such as rate of oral absorption, half-life of elimination, and presence of active metabolites.

Remember also that all of these drugs have adverse effects that are only just beginning to be determined. For example, benzodiazepines with long elimination half-lives (greater than 12 to 24 hours), or those drugs with long-lived active metabolites such as flurazepam, have recently been associated not only with daytime somnolence, but also with an increased risk of hip fractures in the elderly because of more falls. Thus, we should never look on these drugs as totally safe, and we should never prescribe them unless they are indicated. In addition, they should be prescribed in the lowest useful dosage for the shortest length of time, especially in elderly patients.

2. As already noted above, diazepam is metabolized to two active metabolites (*N*-desmethyldiazepam and oxazepam) and then an inactive metabolite (oxazepam glucuronide), whereas lorazepam has only an inactive glucuronide metabolite. Cimetidine will tend to inhibit the P450 enzymes that metabolize diazepam, but not inhibit glucuronyl transferase. Therefore, metabolism of diazepam will be slowed (leading to higher steady-state levels), whereas metabolism of lorazepam will be essentially unchanged (with unchanged steady-state levels). Since steady-state levels are related to both beneficial effects (control of panic attacks) and adverse effects (e.g., somnolence), the implications are obvious.

3. Any alcoholic who is found stuporous must be suspected of having relapsed into drinking. The evaluation of such patients would include measurement of blood or expired breath alcohol concentrations. Assuming the results of these tests were negative, other causes for the stupor must be sought. For example, he might have a subdural hematoma from a fall, meningitis, pneumonia, hypothermia, or a low blood sugar level related to his drinking.

In addition, he has been taking large doses of diazepam for more than a week. In an elderly man, the half-life of diazepam may be as long as 4 days, so that steady-state levels will not be reached for about 4 half-lives (see Fig. 35-1). The presence of alcoholic hepatitis or cirrhosis could slow the metabolism of diazepam even further. No wonder that as he continued to take diazepam at home after his discharge, his serum levels would continue to rise towards the steady-state "plateau" and increasing obtundation would occur.

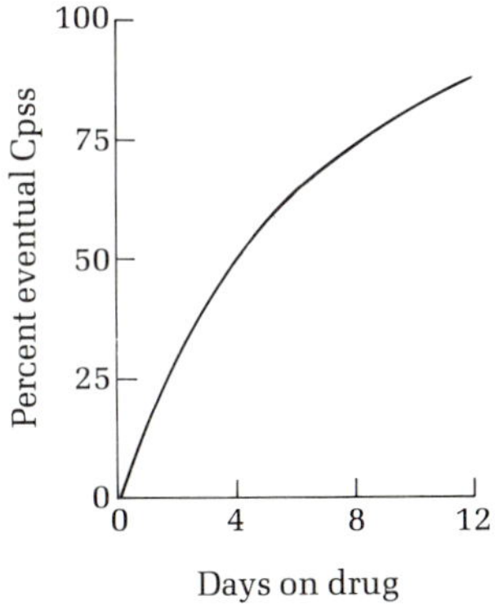

FIG. 35-1. Accumulation of diazepam. Assuming that the drug has an elimination half-life of 4 days, it will have reached only 50% of its eventual steady-state level after one half-life; 75% of its steady-state level after two half-lives; and 87% of its steady-state level after three half-lives.

CHAPTER 36

OTHER SEDATIVE/HYPNOTIC DRUGS

Related Readings

Clark et al: Chapter 24, pp. 260-265; Chapter 26, pp. 286-292
Craig and Stitzel: Chapter 35, pp. 504-511
Gilman et al: Chapter 17, pp. 351-369; Chapter 19, pp. 432-438
Katzung: Chapter 20

Key Concepts

- Properties of secobarbital and barbiturates in general
- Pharmacokinetic and pharmacodynamic differences between secobarbital and phenobarbital
- Pharmacokinetic and pharmacodynamic properties of thiopental

QUESTIONS

1. Six patients were sitting in their physician's waiting room and were comparing their past experiences with a drug called secobarbital. The first patient mentioned that he was taking secobarbital 50 mg orally 3 times daily as a sedative; the second patient mentioned that he was taking secobarbital 50 mg orally 2 times daily to manage his feelings of anxiety; a third

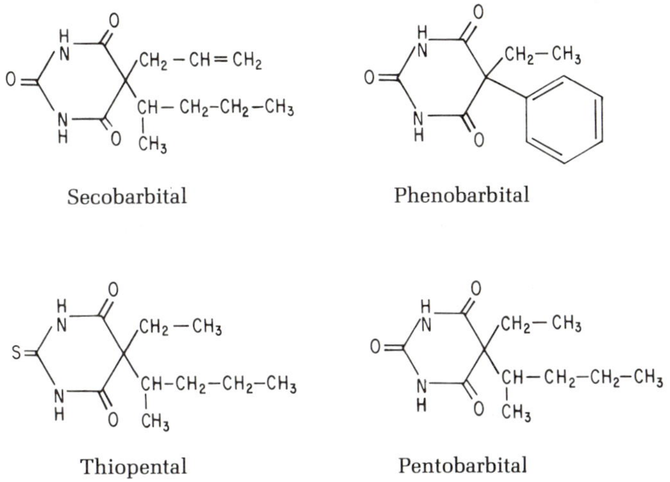

FIG. 36-1. Structures of four barbiturates—secobarbital, phenobarbital, thiopental, and pentobarbital.

3. The intravenous route, of course, results in a rapid elevation of blood levels of thiopental. The drug's high lipid solubility (Fig. 36-1) allows the drug to rapidly cross into the brain and results in a rapid loss of consciousness. In fact, most patients lose consciousness 5 to 30 seconds after the injection begins. This rapid induction of unconsciousness is preferable to the slower inductions achieved with some inhalational agents.

That same high lipid solubility, however, also facilitates a rapid redistribution of the drug from brain and blood into body fat stores and skeletal muscle, so that the loss of consciousness that follows a single bolus is very transient. In fact, the effects of that one intravenous injection only last for about 10 to 20 minutes. The true elimination of thiopental from the body involves biotransformation and excretion of metabolites in the urine. These processes lag hours behind the rapid redistribution that terminates the drug effect but does not eliminate the drug from the body. Administration by slow intravenous drip can produce a state of anesthesia that continues as long as the drug is being given. However, this would not be a good way to maintain anesthesia, since once the surgery was completed, the anesthetic would be very slow to wear off (half-life about 6 hours). In addition, if thiopental levels rise very high, the metabolic routes become saturated and the kinetics of elimination change from first-order to zero-order. From your lectures on kinetics, you will recognize that the "half-life" of elimination under these conditions can be 18 hours or even longer.

CHAPTER 37

ANTIPSYCHOTIC DRUGS

Related Readings

Clark et al: Chapter 24, pp. 250-259
Craig and Stitzel: Chapter 38, pp. 533-543
Gilman et al: Chapter 19, pp. 387-412
Katzung: Chapter 27, pp. 315-324

Key Concepts

- Terminology: minor tranquilizers, major tranquilizers, neuroleptics, antipsychotics
- The dopamine hypothesis of schizophrenia
- Adverse effects of neuroleptic agents

QUESTIONS

1. One of your relatives mentions that he has recently been prescribed a "tranquilizer" and is not sure why. He asks you what type of drug has been prescribed. Do you know?

2. Schizophrenia is one type of psychosis that has been particularly well studied. From these studies has emerged the "dopamine hypothesis" of schizophrenia. What observations led to this hypothesis? Why is one of these observations now almost a self-fulfilling prophecy?

3. Patients receiving the various antipsychotic drugs may develop a number of adverse effects, including dry mouth, difficulty urinating, blurred vision, hypotension, impotence, pseudoparkinsonism, acute bizarre movement disorders (acute dystonic reactions), acute confusion, and even endocrine problems. Over many months, some patients even develop a severe and sometimes irreversible movement disorder known as tardive dyskinesia. How can these drugs designed to be dopaminergic receptor antagonists cause all these problems? Are all of these drugs equally likely to cause all of these adverse reactions?

ANSWERS

1. Many physicians use the term "tranquilizer" loosely to describe to their patients what type of effect they are trying to achieve. Given only that information, it is not possible to know whether the drug was an antipsychotic drug (sometimes called a neuroleptic or "major" tranquilizer) or a sedative-hypnotic drug (such as a benzodiazepine or barbiturate, also known as "minor" tranquilizers). The term "tranquilizer" is sufficiently imprecise that it is probably best to avoid it altogether.

2. The central abnormality in schizophrenia has been ascribed at least partly to an overactivity of dopaminergic pathways in the mesolimbic-frontal system. The following are observations that led to this hypothesis: (1) all antipsychotic drugs currently in use block postsynaptic dopamine receptors; (2) an increase in dopaminergic activity (as in the administration of levodopa for parkinsonism) may result in psychotic side effects; and (3) abuse of sympathomimetic stimulants such as amphetamine often results in paranoid schizophrenia. Most screening programs for identifying antipsychotic drugs are now based on the ability of the potential drug to block dopamine receptors. Thus, the very way we test new drugs for potential antipsychotic effects (testing for dopaminergic blocking effects) serves to guarantee that our newer antipsychotic agents will demonstrate similar pharmacologic properties, at least with respect to dopamine receptors.

3. Although the antipsychotic drugs are presumably effective because they block dopamine receptors in the mesolimbic system, the same action in the tuberoinfundibular system releases prolactin, resulting in galactorrhea and hypogonadism. Blockade of dopamine receptors in the nigrostriatal pathway may produce symptoms of parkinsonism. Many of these antipsychotic drugs also exhibit some ability to block muscarinic receptors, leading to symptoms of dry mouth, blurred vision, delirium, constipation and urinary retention. Blockade of alpha-adrenergic receptors may result in othostatic hypotension, impotence, and failure to ejaculate. Long-term use can lead to a bizarre, chronic movement disorder known as tardive dyskinesia, possibly caused by supersensitivity of dopamine receptors. Antipsychotic drugs also differ in their relative abilities to cause sedation.

There are advantages and disadvantages among the various antipsychotic drugs. Some, like chlorpromazine, are more likely to cause sedation and hypotension. Butyrophenones usually do not cause cardiovascular problems, but they may be associated with an increased risk of acute dystonic reactions. Fluphenazine-like drugs seem to have an increased ability to cause tardive dyskinesias. None of these drugs (or drug classes) is perfect, but their different profiles of side effects may make one drug or one class of drugs preferable in a particular patient.

CHAPTER 38

ANTIDEPRESSANT DRUGS

Related Readings

Clark et al: Chapter 25, pp. 268-274
Craig and Stitzel: Chapter 39
Gilman et al: Chapter 19, pp. 412-432
Katzung: Chapter 28

Key Concepts

- Indications for treatment of depression, adverse effects of tricyclic agents
- Mechanisms of action of various classes of antidepressant drugs

QUESTIONS

1. The 67-year-old woman who lives next door to you has never complained of depression in her life. However, 3 weeks ago her 13-year-old dog died of natural causes and she has been "sad and depressed" ever since. She tells you that she is eating and sleeping normally and is still performing her volunteer work at the library, but she is just "sad" all the time. Her physician has placed her on amitriptyline, and she has noticed that she has become more sleepy and has developed constipation. She has not noticed any change in her sadness. Can you explain all of this?

2. Occasionally the adverse effects caused by one drug result in the development of a new class of drugs which have the "opposite" effect. How did the adverse effects of reserpine lead to the "amine hypothesis" of depression? According to this hypothesis, how do the three broad classes of antidepressant drugs ameliorate depression?

ANSWERS

1. The woman is suffering an understandable loss with the recent death of her pet. Although she is sad and grieving, this would not be characterized as a serious, incapacitating depression. After all, she is eating and sleeping normally and can still carry on her usual daily activities. She probably just needs some time to get over this loss, and specific drug treatment probably would not be beneficial.

However, her physician did start her on amitriptyline, which is from the class of "tricyclic" antidepressants. These drugs often cause sedation and/or anticholinergic effects (e.g., constipation). It is unlikely that this drug will help her, but if it does, no change will be noticed for 2 to 3 weeks at the earliest. At this point, she has demonstrated several adverse reactions with no evidence of beneficial effects—not a good result!

2. A frequent side effect of reserpine (when it was given in large doses to lower blood pressure) was the development of "melancholia" (depression). Since reserpine was known to deplete catecholamines in noradrenergic neurons, it was postulated that depression was caused by failure of adrenergic transmission. All of the drugs used to treat depression help to facilitate adrenergic transmission: (1) the tricyclics block norepinephrine re-uptake by nerve terminals; (2) the monoamine oxidase inhibitors block nor-epinephrine breakdown in nerve terminals; and (3) adrenergic agonists like amphetamine, although a poor choice, are sometimes effective in depression.

CHAPTER 39

ANTIPARKINSONIAN DRUGS

Related Readings

Clark et al: Chapter 12, pp. 121-126
Craig and Stitzel: Chapter 41
Gilman et al: Chapter 21
Katzung: Chapter 26

Key Concepts

- Pathophysiology of Parkinson's disease, common drugs used for that disorder
- Adverse effects of L-dopa

QUESTIONS

1. One of your elderly neighbors has a movement disorder characterized by slow movements, rigidity, a constant tremor, and a slow, shuffling gait. He recently saw his physician, and came home with prescriptions for oral benztropine mesylate and large doses of levodopa. What disease does the physician think that your neighbor has? Why were these two drugs chosen?

2. The patient above develops anorexia, nausea, and vomiting soon after treatment is begun. He feels a little dizzy when he stands suddenly, and he wonders if his new medications are causing any of these problems. He feels that the drugs have not helped his "brain," but are harming his "body." How would you respond to these concerns of the patient?

ANSWERS

1. The symptoms of abnormal movement mentioned here are typical of parkinsonism. Levodopa (L-dopa) was prescribed because it is bioavailable when given orally, and is able to cross the blood-brain barrier. Once in the brain, it is converted by dopa-decarboxylase to dopamine, and thereby helps restore dopaminergic tone in the basal ganglia.

Parkinson's disease is thought to represent an imbalance between dopaminergic tone (too little) and cholinergic tone (relatively too much). Benztropine mesylate has anticholinergic (antimuscarinic) effects, is bioavailable when taken orally, and is able to cross the blood-brain barrier. Therefore, it is often a useful adjunct when given with L-dopa.

2. Anorexia, nausea and vomiting are common side effects of L-dopa. After absorption, much of the L-dopa is converted to dopamine in the periphery of the body, before the L-dopa enters the central nervous system. These symptoms are thought to be caused by the dopamine that is formed peripherally, and they can be reproduced by administering dopamine intravenously. Since we want L-dopa to be converted to dopamine in the brain but not in the rest of the body, it would be useful to inhibit the enzyme dopa-decarboxylase peripherally, but not in the brain.

Fortunately, a drug exists with just these useful properties. Carbidopa blocks the enzyme dopa-decarboxylase, thereby blocking the conversion of dopa to dopamine. However, it does not cross the blood-brain barrier. The net effects are to reduce the amount of dopamine formed peripherally and to increase the amount of L-dopa available for redistribution into the central nervous system. Thus, the oral dose of L-dopa can be substantially reduced when carbidopa is also prescribed.

CHAPTER 40

ANTI-EPILEPTIC DRUGS

Related Readings

Clark et al: Chapter 28
Craig and Stitzel: Chapter 40
Gilman et al: Chapter 20
Katzung: Chapter 22

Key Concepts

- Emergency management of severe grand mal seizures
- Actions of phenytoin, therapeutic serum concentrations

QUESTIONS

1. A middle-aged woman with a prior history of epilepsy is brought to your emergency room while she is experiencing a series of grand mal seizures, one leading into the next. This is a dangerous condition known as *status epilepticus*. What drug could you give rapidly via the intravenous route that should interrupt these seizures within only a few minutes? How long will this beneficial effect last? Is this drug useful via the oral route for chronic control of these seizures?

2. A 14-year-old girl has taken oral phenytoin 300 mg per day for the last several years to control her grand mal seizures. She has taken the drug reliably, has had therapeutic plasma levels (hers run 14 to 17 μg/ml), and has averaged less than one seizure per year. During the last month she has had three grand mal seizures—a sharp increase for her. Her plasma level was checked, and the phenytoin level was only 3 μg/ml—definitely in the subtherapeutic range. What possibilities would you consider for this sudden change in plasma level and clinical effect?

ANSWERS

1. The drug of choice for this situation would be intravenous diazepam (or lorazepam, a very similar benzodiazepine). It may be given as a slow intravenous push and is effective after just 1 to 2 minutes. It rapidly attains high blood and brain levels because of its lipid solubility. Although diazepam has a half-life of elimination of 24 hours or more, its antiseizure effects last for only 15 to 30 minutes because of rapid redistribution. However, this period of seizure control gives you time to administer a longer-acting drug such as phenobarbital or phenytoin. Status epilepticus is the only form or complication of epilepsy in which diazepam is of proven value.

Oral diazepam as chronic therapy is not useful because the serum levels necessary to control seizures also cause excessive sedation. Phenytoin or phenobarbital can be given chronically for long-term control because the dose-response curves for seizure control (Fig. 40-1) and sedation (or other toxicity) are more widely separated (i.e., a larger therapeutic index).

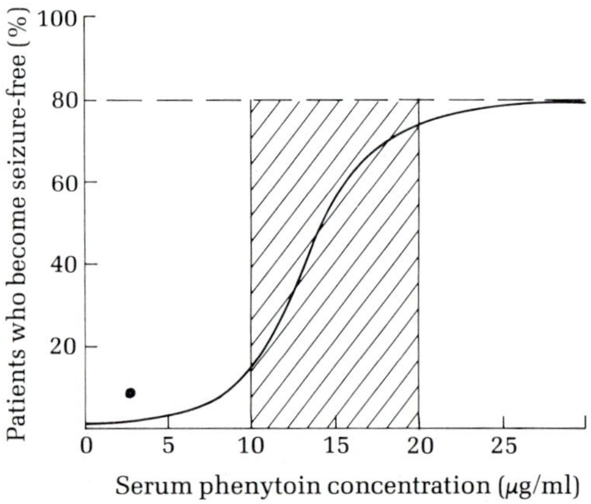

FIG. 40-1. Representative concentration-effect curve for a group of patients with grand mal epilepsy treated with phenytoin. Notice that a few patients become seizure-free with serum concentrations as low as 5 μg/ml. However, most patients experience improvement in their seizures when serum levels are between 10 and 20 μg/ml (the recognized therapeutic range). A few patients become seizure-free when the levels are above 20 μg/ml, and some patients will improve but not become seizure-free even at high serum levels. Although not shown on this figure, few patients will experience dose-related side effects at levels less than 20 μg/ml.

2. The most likely reason for the sudden drop in plasma levels and the loss of the clinical benefit of the drug is patient noncompliance. She has stopped taking the drug or greatly reduced her dosage. As a teenager, she is aware of the stigma of seizures, and she may be reluctant to be seen taking her medication in school. Another possibility is that she is suffering from one of the side effects of this drug—gingival hyperplasia, or excessive thickening of her gums. This may be particularly traumatic for teenagers. She may be more willing to endure increased seizures than to suffer this unpleasant side effect.

Other less likely explanations include switching the brand of phenytoin, with a sudden decrease in oral bioavailability (very unlikely given current FDA standards in this area), or a marked increase in the rate of metabolism (perhaps caused by enzyme induction by a new medication recently added). A detailed history, and possibly peak and trough serum levels, would help you evaluate which of these explanations is the correct one.

SECTION SEVEN

DRUGS USED FOR CARDIOVASCULAR DISEASES

CHAPTER 41

DIGITALIS

Related Readings

Clark et al: Chapter 34
Craig and Stitzel: Chapter 24
Gilman et al: Chapter 30
Katzung: Chapter 12

Key Concepts

- Effects of digoxin on cardiac impulse formation and conduction, characteristics of arrhythmias induced by digoxin
- Indications for prescribing digoxin, errors in drug use

QUESTIONS

1. A "classic" arrhythmia seen in some patients with digoxin toxicity is paroxysmal atrial tachycardia combined with atrioventricular (AV) block. What do both of these phrases mean in rough electrophysiologic terms? How does understanding this arrhythmia help you understand the primary effects of this drug on impulse formation and conduction in the heart?

2. You admit a patient to your coronary care unit who is recovering from an acute myocardial infarction. He has been receiving oral digoxin 0.25 mg daily for the last 3 years to help control some "fluid on his lungs" that occurred 3 years ago during an episode of pneumonia. You write an order to continue the digoxin every morning. In addition, you request that a plasma sample be sent by the nurse the next morning to check the level. That afternoon, the plasma digoxin concentration drawn at 9:30 AM returns at 5 ng/ml. You are stat paged by the CCU nurse to come see your patient who has a toxic level. Your patient remains asymptomatic. What is your assessment of this situation?

ANSWERS

1. The paroxysmal atrial tachycardia (a sustained atrial tachycardia often triggered by an abnormal pacemaker and sustained by reentrant conduction) is secondary to the predominant effect of digoxin on the atria, namely, a shortening of the refractory period. The resting membrane potential becomes more depolarized as a result of inhibition of the sodium pump (Na-K-ATPase), there is a marked shortening of the action potential, and oscillatory after-depolarizations (caused by abnormal increases in intracellular calcium) may occur. All these factors contribute to atrial premature beats and atrial tachycardia. Thus, one effect of digoxin is to speed up pacemaker activity in tissues that are not usually responsible for initiating the heartbeat.

Paradoxically, within the atrioventricular (AV) node the same biochemical events (and other indirect effects on the vagus) tend to increase the refractory period and decrease conduction velocity through the AV node. If an impulse from the atria tries to get through the AV node, it may hit the node during its prolonged refractory period and not be conducted—atrioventricular block. Thus, increased AV block is also a characteristic digoxin effect.

In short, "classic" digitalis-related arrhythmias often combine increased automaticity and increased AV block to produce arrhythmias such as paroxysmal atrial tachycardia with AV block. These arrhythmias may be predicted once you understand the effects of this drug on impulse formation and conduction.

2. Many patients receive digoxin chronically even when they do not have a good reason for receiving the drug. Recognized indications include slowing the ventricular response during atrial fibrillation and treating congestive heart failure that has not responded to diuretics. This patient probably never needed digoxin in the first place—the "fluid on his lung" during one episode of pneumonia was not a sufficient reason to prescribe it, and there was no reason to continue the drug for 3 years. In some studies, up to 45% of patients receiving digoxin chronically did not have a recognized indication for receiving the drug.

The pharmacokinetics of digoxin are unusual in that it has a very large volume of distribution because of extensive binding to sites in the heart and other tissues. The redistribution from plasma to tissue sites takes time, which accounts for an unusually long alpha-phase of the plasma concentration-time curve. In other words, plasma levels obtained in the 6 to 8 hours following a dose of digoxin do not accurately reflect the steady-state plasma or tissue levels, and therefore blood samples should not be drawn before the alpha-phase is complete. This blood sample was drawn prematurely before redistribution was completed, and the result was nearly impossible to interpret. In addition, there was no clear reason for the drug level to have been ordered in the first place. The diagnosis of digoxin toxicity should be made based on the patient's symptoms, signs, and electrocardiogram.

Finally, digoxin would be a good drug to avoid in the peri-infarction period unless there is a specific reason to give it, since it may increase the risk of arrhythmias. In short, this patient illustrates a few of the common mistakes associated with the irrational prescribing of digoxin and the irrational ordering of digoxin blood levels.

CHAPTER 42

INOTROPIC AND CHRONOTROPIC DRUGS

Related Readings

Clark et al: Chapter 34
Craig and Stitzel: Chapter 24
Gilman et al: Chapter 30
Katzung: Chapter 12

Key Concepts

- Significance of bradycardia, choice of chronotropic agents
- Drugs that produce acute inotropic effects

QUESTIONS

1. You are called by a nurse to see a patient who has a pulse of 30 BPM. You obtain an ECG that reveals sinus rhythm (a sinus bradycardia). Should you treat this patient? If you do, what types of drugs could be used to help accelerate the rate of firing of the sinoatrial node?

2. One of your patients is in the coronary care unit recovering from an acute myocardial infarction. His blood pressure is barely adequate (90/60 mm Hg), he is slightly tachycardic (pulse 150 BPM), and hemodynamic data reveal he has a low cardiac output, normal vascular resistance, and adequate filling pressures. You wish to administer a drug that will rapidly improve the contractility of the heart without having a marked effect on heart rate. What drugs are available to you for this purpose? How do they work?

ANSWERS

1. Before instituting any drug therapy, the patient should be carefully evaluated. There may be a perfectly valid reason for a slow pulse (e.g., an athlete in top shape may have a pulse of 30 BPM; Bjorn Borg apparently had a resting pulse of around 32 BPM).

However, if examination of the patient reveals that this pulse rate is pathologically slow and associated with symptoms (such as hypotension or inadequate cardiac output), then treatment is indicated. The drug of first choice would be atropine, a muscarinic receptor blocker. Atropine should help speed up the heart rate if excessive vagal tone is partially responsible.

If atropine fails to work, then a beta-1 adrenergic receptor agonist may be needed. Isoproterenol is the prototypical nonspecific beta-receptor agonist that is most commonly used in this situation. Thus the rate of firing of the sinoatrial node may be accelerated either by blocking muscarinic receptor stimulation or by giving beta-1 receptor agonists.

2. You are looking for a drug that has predominantly inotropic effects with minimal chronotropic effects. Accelerating the heart rate in this situation would likely cause increased myocardial oxygen consumption, which could worsen the patient's myocardial ischemia. Two prototype drugs could be used to improve the contractility of the heart without greatly increasing the heart rate. The first of these is dobutamine, a selective beta-1 agonist. It is not clear why dobutamine usually has so little effect on heart rate when similar drugs such as dopamine have prominent effects on heart rate. It has been suggested that since dobutamine is a racemic mixture, the different stereoisomers may have somewhat opposing effects.

The other class of drugs that exhibit acute inotropic effects are the so-called bipyridines (amrinone and milrinone). They appear to act by increasing calcium influx into myocardial cells and by inhibiting phosphodiesterase to conserve intracellular cAMP. These effects improve cardiac muscle cell contractility without greatly increasing the heart rate.

Both intravenous dobutamine and intravenous amrinone have been used to increase the contractility of the heart in this serious situation. As you recall from basic physiology, you are trying the shift the heart onto a better Starling curve. It is likely that in the future better and more specific positive inotropic agents will become available.

CHAPTER 43

NITRATES AND METHYLXANTHINES

Related Readings

Clark et al: Chapters 30 and 40
Craig and Stitzel: Chapter 25, and Chapter 72, pp. 1014-1017
Gilman et al: Chapter 25, and Chapter 33, pp. 806-816
Katzung: Chapters 11 and 18

Key Concepts

- Drug of choice for angina pectoris, mechanism of action of nitroglycerin
- Pharmacologic effects of caffeine, structural similarities with theophylline

QUESTIONS

1. You have a 75-year-old uncle with classic angina pectoris brought on by exertion. He claims that he can prevent getting chest pains by avoiding walking up stairs. On the other hand, if his pain occurs, he sits down and places one prescribed tablet under his tongue. This tablet rapidly dissolves, creating a local burning sensation. He then notices a headache and a flushed sensation, and 2 minutes later his chest pain and pressure resolve. What drug did he take? How did it cause all of these effects?

2. A medical student stays up all night to study for an examination. During the night, he drinks 11 cups of regular coffee. He begins to notice a slight tremor, rapid and sometimes irregular pulse, and an increased urge to urinate. What ingredient in the coffee caused these effects? What other effects might have occurred without his noticing? Is coffee ever used as a drug to achieve these effects?

ANSWERS

1. Your uncle takes glyceryl trinitrate (trinitroglycerin, nitroglycerin, GTN) sublingually. It is not a particularly pleasant drug to take, but it is preferable to the pain of angina. The burning sensation under the tongue is caused by intense local vasodilatation. The headache is presumably a result of dilation of the meningeal arteries, and the flush is the result of dilation of cutaneous blood vessels.

The desired effect, resolution of chest pain and pressure, is probably related to two effects. First, ventricular work and oxygen consumption are reduced. Preload is reduced because of dilation of large veins (venodilatation), and afterload is reduced because of reduced ventricular volume and reduced arterial pressure (mild vasodilatation). Second, myocardial oxygen delivery may be increased in some patients by vasodilatation of portions of the coronary circulation.

Although the relative contributions of these two mechanisms of action are not completely resolved, it remains firmly established that nitroglycerin is the drug of choice to relieve the acute pain or pressure of angina. In addition, the drug may be taken before a stressful activity to preclude the development of angina.

2. The student is experiencing the effects of mild caffeine poisoning. The tremor is a result of a central stimulant effect. Caffeine also increases the rate and contractility of the heart, which may result in tachyarrhythmias and the sense of palpitations. Its diuretic effect is caused by an inhibition of renal tubular sodium reabsorption.

He may not have noticed a mild stimulation of respiration, bronchodilation, increased secretion of gastric acid, or better functioning of his skeletal muscles.

Coffee is widely used as a "recreational" drug to achieve some of these effects, and the medical student was seeking its stimulant effects on the central nervous system. Caffeine is rarely prescribed or used by physicians today. However, a closely related drug—theophylline—is often prescribed for its bronchodilatory effects in patients with obstructive lung disease (Fig. 43-1). Not surprisingly, many of the side effects of theophylline are similar to those of caffeine.

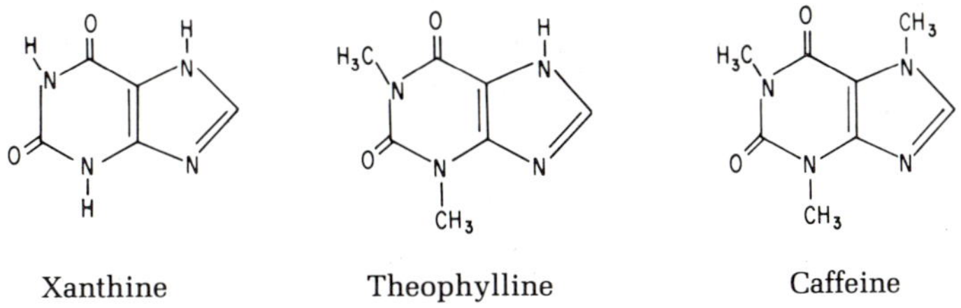

FIG. 43-1. Structures of caffeine, theophylline, and xanthine. Notice how similar the two methylxanthines are in chemical structure.

CHAPTER 44

DIURETIC AGENTS I

Related Readings

Clark et al: Chapter 38
Craig and Stitzel: Chapter 21
Gilman et al: Chapter 36
Katzung: Chapter 14

Key Concepts

- Metabolic effects of thiazide diuretics
- Determinants of timing and extent of diuresis induced by furosemide

QUESTIONS

1. A 65-year-old man had mild diabetes (no treatment required) and mild congestive heart failure, with slight fluid retention and ankle edema. His doctor prescribed oral hydrochlorothiazide (50 mg every morning) to help eliminate the ankle edema. Over the next 2 weeks the patient noticed that his ankles were slightly less puffy, but he also noticed that he felt a bit weaker, he developed an acute episode of gout in his large toe, and he noted the new onset of polyuria and polydipsia (frequent drinking and urinating). Are these symptoms related to the initiation of diuretic therapy?

2. A patient with severe congestive heart failure and fluid retention is being treated by a team of three interns. On day one, the first intern prescribes furosemide 40 mg intravenously. A diuresis of approximately 700 ml ensues over the next 4 hours. Two days later, the second intern prescribes furosemide 40 mg orally. Several days later probenecid is started to reduce chronic hyperuricemia, and a few days after that the third intern also prescribes furosemide 40 mg orally. How will the effects of furosemide prescribed by the second and third interns compare to the diuresis induced by the first intravenous dose?

ANSWERS

1. The hydrochlorothiazide seemed to be having its desired effect in relieving edema, since the patient's ankles were slightly less puffy. Unfortunately, several adverse effects appear to have developed as well. The attack of acute gout was probably brought on by hydrocholorothiazide-induced hyperuricemia. Possibly related to contracted extracellular fluid volume, reabsorption of uric acid in the renal tubules was increased, with resultant development of hyperuricemia. An acute episode of gout ensued.

The diuretic also worsened the patient's diabetes either by producing pancreatitis (rare), or by decreasing insulin secretion by beta cells of the pancreas (more common). Finally, the patient's general weakness could be related to diuretic-induced hypokalemia. It is important to remember these common metabolic effects associated with the use of thiazide diuretics.

2. Furosemide is a "loop diuretic" that is often effective at inducing a diuresis even when a thiazide diuretic fails. However, the oral bioavailability of furosemide is only about 61%. Since it was given in the same dose orally as intravenously, its oral use will result in a smaller diuretic effect. One might anticipate a total diuresis of about 61% of 700 ml, or about 420 ml. In addition, the diuresis that follows oral administration begins later and persists longer than that seen following intravenous administration, since the appearance of the drug in the serum and the urine is relatively delayed by the process of absorption. Thus, the second dose of furosemide given orally should result in a smaller diuresis, with delayed onset and more prolonged duration.

In the meantime, probenecid has been added to the drug regimen. Both probenecid and furosemide are actively secreted into the renal tubule, and when present together will compete for the same transport mechanism. Since furosemide must be present in the tubular fluid to exert its diuretic effect, probenecid will slow the rate of delivery of furosemide into tubular fluid. The net result would be a delayed and prolonged diuresis when furosemide is given with probenecid, but no change in the total amount of the diuresis.

CHAPTER 45

DIURETIC AGENTS II

Related Readings

Clark et al: Chapter 38
Craig and Stitzel: Chapter 21
Gilman et al: Chapter 36
Katzung: Chapter 14

Key Concepts

- Sites of action of furosemide and metolazone
- Differences between thiazide diuretics and potassium-sparing diuretics

QUESTIONS

1. A patient with severe congestive heart failure and fluid retention gradually required more and more furosemide to produce a diuresis, finally requiring doses of 400 mg by mouth. In an effort to potentiate this diuresis, the physician continued the furosemide and added a simultaneous dose of metolazone. What is the rationale of adding a "weaker" diuretic to a "strong" diuretic in this situation?

2. A 65-year-old patient takes digoxin to control his atrial fibrillation. When he develops hypertension, his doctor prescribes hydrochlorothiazide 50 mg by mouth twice daily. The patient takes his blood pressure at home, and notices that this medication seems to control his blood pressure well. However, during his next clinic visit, his doctor obtains a blood test and then prescribes a second diuretic, triamterene. This does not make sense to him, because his blood pressure seemed to be well controlled. On his third visit, after another blood test is obtained, his doctor discontinues both diuretics, and prescribes yet a third—Dyazide™. What is the meaning of these changes in prescriptions?

ANSWERS

1. One of the reasons for this patient's becoming refractory to the effects of large doses of the loop diuretic, furosemide, may be that his kidneys are simply not delivering much sodium and chloride to the loop of Henle because of extensive proximal reabsorption. The thiazide diuretics, such as metolazone, prevent the reabsorption of salt and water in the proximal tubule and in the early segments of the distal tubule. When only a thiazide is given, the effects on the proximal tubule are usually not important, since absorption of salt and water in the loop of Henle can compensate.

However, when furosemide blocks salt and water reabsorption in the loop of Henle, then the effect of thiazides in the proximal tubule becomes important. In the presence of metolazone, more salt and water is delivered to the loop of Henle, where furosemide prevents its reabsorption. This salt and water is passed along to the distal tubule, where again the thiazide helps prevent its reabsorption. Thus, giving these two diuretics together makes sense based upon the different sites of action of the two diuretics. A "weak" diuretic may actually greatly potentiate the diuretic effect of a "strong" diuretic.

2. The first diuretic prescribed was hydrochlorothiazide. The blood test taken probably indicated a low serum potassium level (hypokalemia) secondary to the potassium "wasting" effect of the thiazide. This could be a problem, especially in a patient also taking digoxin.

Triamterene is a potassium-sparing diuretic. The three commonly used agents (triamterene, amiloride, and spironolactone) all act in the cortical collecting tubule to antagonize the effects of aldosterone, which itself promotes loss of potassium in exchange for reabsorption of sodium. Triamterene appears to directly inhibit sodium transport within the collecting tubule. It was prescribed not so much for its diuretic effect or its weak antihypertensive effect as for its ability to conserve potassium and prevent hypokalemia.

Dyazide(TM) is the trade name for a fixed ratio combination of hydrochlorothiazide (25 mg) and triamterene (50 mg). It is more expensive, but it has the advantage that the patient can take his daily dose of two diuretics in one capsule. The increased cost may be offset by the advantage of increased compliance.

CHAPTER 46

ANTIHYPERTENSIVE AGENTS I

Related Readings

Clark et al: Chapter 18
Craig and Stitzel: Chapter 22
Gilman et al: Chapter 32
Katzung: Chapter 10

Key Concepts

- Mechanisms sustaining systemic hypertension; mechanisms of action of antihypertensive drugs
- Difference between primary (essential) and secondary hypertension

QUESTIONS

1. Consider two "hypertensive" patients. The first is a 22-year-old man with a mean arterial pressure of 120 mm Hg (blood pressure 200/80 mm Hg), a cardiac output of 20 L/minute, and a systemic vascular resistance of 480 dyne sec cm^{-5} (normal resistance in these units is 700 to 1200). The second patient is a 67-year-old man with the same mean arterial pressure of 120 mm Hg (blood pressure 160/100 mm Hg), but with a cardiac output of 3 L/minute and a systemic vascular resistance of 3200 dyne sec cm^{-5}. What type of patients do you think these two men represent? What do they illustrate about two basic mechanisms for producing systemic hypertension?

2. A 23-year-old woman with chronic asthma has her first physical examination in several years because it is required by her employer. The physician notices that her blood pressure is 180/120 mm Hg in the right arm, and about the same in her left arm. When he palpates diminished femoral pulses, he uses a larger blood pressure cuff and finds that the pressures in her legs are only 90/50 mm Hg. In addition, he hears a harsh systolic murmur across the precordium, and he hears it even better when he listens to her lungs from the back. Because of the severe degree of hypertension, the physician prescribes usual dosages of hydrochlorothiazide and propranolol. What do you think of this overall approach to her hypertension?

ANSWERS

1. Both patients were clearly hypertensive at the time their blood pressures were measured, if we define "normal" blood pressure as 120/80 mm Hg. The hemodynamic parameters of the first patient suggest that he is a healthy young adult who has been exercising vigorously. Vigorous exercise is associated with an increased cardiac output (in this case, increased from 5 L/minute to 20 L/minute), increased systolic blood pressure, no increase in diastolic blood pressure, increase in mean arterial pressure, and a marked fall in systemic vascular resistance. Thus, the hypertension here is associated with a large increase in cardiac output, and a drop in resistance. This is a normal response to vigorous exercise, and requires no treatment. In fact, treatment would be harmful.

The elderly gentleman has hypertension generated in an entirely different way. He probably has some type of heart disease with a reduced cardiac output (3 L/minute). His elevated blood pressure and decreased cardiac output are associated with a dramatically increased systemic vascular resistance (3200 dyne sec cm^{-5}), probably secondary to increased levels of norepinephrine and angiotensin II. In this patient, "afterload reduction" with a vasodilator to decrease this resistance might well reduce the blood pressure slightly, and might even result in a slight increase in cardiac output.

These two patients illustrate that elevated mean arterial pressure can result from increases in either cardiac output or systemic vascular resistance. Therefore, it is not surprising that most antihypertensive agents reduce blood pressure by reducing systemic vascular resistance, whereas others reduce blood pressure by reducing the cardiac output. Some antihypertensive drugs work by way of both mechanisms.

2. This young woman has a coarctation of the aorta. This congenital narrowing of the aorta usually occurs distal to the origin of the left subclavian artery, and thus the blood pressure measured in the arms is greater than that measured in the legs. The femoral arteries, when palpated, often show diminished pulsations that may be delayed relative to the radial arteries. Also, the aortic narrowing results in a flow murmur best heard from the back. Such a condition should be detected in childhood, but it may be first detected in early adulthood as well.

Coarctation of the aorta is one of many examples of secondary hypertension—hypertension caused by a specific primary pathologic condition. Various populations of hypertensive patients have been shown to have secondary hypertension in from 5% to 35% of cases. The definitive treatment in this case would not be drug therapy, but rather surgical correction of the abnormality in the aorta.

It is important to rule out secondary hypertension before beginning treatment for primary, idiopathic, or "essential" hypertension. Other causes of secondary hypertension include renovascular disease, hyperaldosteronism, pheochromocytoma, and ingestion of certain drugs. The important point to remember is that specific causes of secondary hypertension usually respond best to specific treatments when they are available.

CHAPTER 47

ANTIHYPERTENSIVE AGENTS II

Related Readings

Clark et al: Chapter 18
Craig and Stitzel: Chapter 22
Gilman et al: Chapter 31
Katzung: Chapter 10

Key Concepts

- Importance of side effects of antihypertensive agents; individualization of therapy
- Rational use of antihypertensive agents in episodes of "hypertensive crisis"

QUESTIONS

1. A 45-year-old man with documented hypertension (blood pressure 160/100 mm Hg on two consecutive office visits) and mild stable angina has a negative workup for reversible lesions, and is given a diagnosis of essential hypertension. He is given hydralazine 50 mg by mouth four times daily. His blood pressure begins to decrease over several days, but after 10 days his blood pressure is back to 160/100 mm Hg. In addition, his episodes of angina have become a bit more frequent. Why has this drug failed to control his hypertension?

2. A 65-year-old man is admitted to the emergency room complaining of a tearing, sharp pain between his shoulder blades. His blood pressure is 190/130 mm Hg, pulse is 120 BPM, and his chest x-ray shows a widened mediastinal shadow. An angiogram confirms the diagnosis of a dissection of his thoracic aorta. Is this a hypertensive crisis? Would you try to lower his blood pressure with drugs? If so, which drugs would you choose, and why?

ANSWERS

1. Hydralazine is a directly-acting vasodilator. It is often impossible to maintain a long-term stable decrease in blood pressure using this type of drug alone. The abrupt initial fall in blood pressure on starting therapy is sensed by the baroreceptors that activate the sympathetic nervous system. This reflex would then produce an increase in heart rate and an attempt to induce sympathetically mediated vasoconstriction.

Also, the kidneys would begin to produce more renin because of decreased renal blood flow and sympathetic activation. This would lead to increased production of angiotensin II, causing increased vasoconstriction. In addition, secretion of aldosterone would increase, leading to salt and water retention. Thus, the body would "escape" from the antihypertensive effects of hydralazine by increasing vasoconstriction, fluid retention, and the heart rate.

These escape mechanisms could be prevented by simultaneous treatment with both a beta-blocker and a diuretic. In fact, use of vasodilators is recommended only as "third line" therapy, if treatment with both a diuretic and a beta-blocker do not lower the blood pressure sufficiently.

Finally, vasodilators can worsen angina when given to patients with ischemic heart disease. The increased chronotropic and inotropic state of the heart results in increased myocardial oxygen consumption, which can obviously result in greater cardiac ischemia. Thus, this type of drug should be used with caution in patients with ischemic heart disease.

2. Any serious medical condition caused or exacerbated by increased blood pressure constitutes a hypertensive crisis. In this case, the patient's aortic dissection is definitely a life-threatening emergency made worse by his elevated blood pressure. The blood pressure must be reduced quickly, but in a controlled fashion.

However, reducing the blood pressure alone is not sufficient for this patient. For example, if intravenous nitroprusside (a direct vasodilator) with excellent minute-to-minute control) were used, the blood pressure would fall in a controlled fashion, but there would be a reflex tachycardia and an increased inotropic state resulting in increased shearing forces in the aorta (dP/dt). Thus, if nitroprusside is used, a beta-blocker must be given as well (preferably first). Other alternatives that lower blood pressure and blunt the increased myocardial response would include intravenous labetolol (a combined alpha- and beta-receptor blocker) or trimethaphan (a ganglionic blocker).

You can see that the choice of antihypertensive medication is often dictated not only by the direct antihypertensive effects of the drugs themselves, but also by the mechanisms of action of the drugs, their "side effects" (other pharmacologic effects), and other medical conditions present in the patient.

CHAPTER 48

ANTI-ARRHYTHMIC AGENTS I

Related Readings

Clark et al: Chapter 35
Craig and Stitzel: Chapter 27
Gilman et al: Chapter 31
Katzung: Chapter 13

Key Concepts

- Drugs useful in preventing ventricular tachyarrhythmias; properties and adverse effects
- Use of beta-blockers as antiarrhythmic agents; adverse effects of beta-blockers
- Rational use of anti-arrhythmic drugs; potential for worsening arrhythmias

QUESTIONS

1. A 50-year-old man is admitted to the coronary care unit with symptoms and ECG findings suggesting an acute myocardial infarction. His blood pressure is 120/80 mm Hg and his pulse is 80 BPM. His heart monitor reveals many ventricular premature beats (VPB) as well. Should he be treated with an anti-arrhythmic agent? If so, how do you choose which one to use?

2. After 1 week, the patient described above is ready to leave the coronary care unit and be transferred to the floor. His lidocaine infusion was successful, and he did not experience any serious arrhythmias. He is on no medications, and feels well although a bit tired. His cardiac monitor reveals occasional VPB, but no severe ectopy (e.g., runs of ventricular tachycardia). In addition, he has no evidence of congestive heart failure. Are any anti-arrhythmic drugs indicated at this point?

ANSWERS

1. In the hours immediately following his heart attack, this patient has a significant chance of developing a potentially lethal ventricular tachyarrhythmia (e.g., ventricular tachycardia or ventricular fibrillation). To prevent such an occurrence, he should receive an appropriate anti-arrhythmic drug—provided that such a drug is safe, and would not cause or worsen other cardiac problems (e.g., heart block, congestive heart failure, hypotension).

The drug that best meets these requirements of efficacy and safety is lidocaine, a Type IB anti-arrhythmic agent. Lidocaine is quite effective in suppressing ventricular premature beats (VPB) and preventing the development of the ventricular arrhythmias in this situation. Because lidocaine does not have strong negative inotropic effects or effects on normal conduction, it is quite unlikely to cause or exacerbate atrioventricular block, bradycardia, congestive heart failure, or hypotension.

Other Type I agents such as procainamide and disopyramide (Type IA agents) are probably as effective as lidocaine in this situation. However, because both of these drugs have strong negative inotropic effects and effects on normal conduction, they are more likely to cause atrioventricular block, hypotension, or congestive heart failure. Thus, lidocaine seems to have the best benefit/risk profile of the commonly used drugs that can be given intravenously, and that are effective in preventing ventricular tachyarrhythmias. If lidocaine fails to work in a particular patient, then a reassessment of risks and benefits may make it appropriate to infuse procainamide, since now its greater risks may be worth taking.

When used in this manner, lidocaine is infused intravenously for 1 to 3 days, until the risk of the patient developing these arrhythmias has dropped sufficiently that the potential benefits of the drug no longer outweigh the potential risks.

2. Patients who have sustained a myocardial infarction are at increased risk during the next year of sustaining either (electrical) sudden death or a subsequent myocardial infarction. This appears to be true even in patients who exhibit neither severe ventricular ectopy after their infarction, nor congestive heart failure.

Several recently completed studies have demonstrated that various beta-receptor blockers (including timolol, propranolol, and metoprolol) can reduce these two risks when given to patients who have sustained a myocardial infarction. Although the mechanism of these preventive effects is not entirely clear, presumably at least part of the protective effect is mediated by the anti-arrhythmic effects of this class of drugs, which in turn are related to their adrenergic receptor blocking properties.

At present, it is not clear whether all patients who have had a heart attack and who do not have a contraindication (severe asthma, heart block, congestive failure) should receive a beta-blocker. Certainly beta-blockers have common and sometimes severe side effects. Efforts are now underway to determine which subset of patients who have had recent heart attacks would benefit most from treatment with beta-blockers.

Remember that learning when to use these drugs rationally is just as important as learning the basic pharmacologic properties of these drugs. For example, consider a different patient recovering from a large myocardial infarction, who has malignant but asymptomatic ventricular ectopy on a 24-hour recording, as well as moderately severe congestive heart failure. This combination has a bad prognosis, with definite increased risk of electrical sudden death during the next year. Nevertheless, it is not obvious that all such patients should receive antiarrhythmic drugs. Studies have not shown that giving this type of patient such drugs increases survival, whereas other studies have shown that perhaps 10% of such patients will actually have their arrhythmias worsened by drug therapy.

CHAPTER 49

ANTI-ARRHYTHMIC AGENTS II

Related Readings

Clark et al: Chapter 35
Craig and Stitzel: Chapter 27
Gilman et al: Chapter 31
Katzung: Chapter 13

Key Concepts

- Therapies for slowing or converting paroxysmal atrial tachycardia
- Interactions between beta-blockers and calcium entry blockers

QUESTIONS

1. A 25-year-old woman comes to the emergency room complaining of palpitations and dizziness. During the examination, she displays signs of anxiety, her blood pressure is 90/60 mm Hg, and her pulse is 180 BPM and regular. Her ECG reveals a paroxysmal atrial tachycardia (PAT). She tells you that she has no history of heart disease, although she has had to come to emergency rooms twice before with the same problem. On both occasions, the arrhythmia was treated with an intravenous drug. How would you proceed?

2. In an effort to control her arrhythmia, the patient described above received several doses of intravenous propranolol. These doses neither slowed the arrhythmia, nor converted it to normal sinus rhythm. At this point, she complains of being even more dizzy. Her blood pressure drops to 80/50 mm Hg, and her pulse remains 180 BPM and regular. The emergency room physician recommends giving her a standard intravenous dose of verapamil, and that is done. Her blood pressure begins to drop sharply, and then her rhythm changes to asystole. What happened?

ANSWERS

1. This episode of paroxysmal atrial tachycardia is associated with moderately severe symptoms (palpitations, hypotension) but not acutely life-threatening problems (e.g., shock, severe angina). Thus, one should consider trying to convert the arrhythmia to normal sinus rhythm or slowing the ventricular response over the next few *minutes*. It would probably not be appropriate to either watch and wait for the arrhythmia to spontaneously stop, nor to proceed with immediate DC cardioversion (works quickly, usually effective, but potentially more painful in a conscious patient and dangerous).

The anti-arrhythmic drug most likely to act within several minutes to convert this arrhythmia to normal sinus rhythm is verapamil. This drug, from the class known as calcium entry blockers, will convert a high percentage (perhaps 85%) of such patients to normal sinus rhythm after one or two doses, delivered over 15 minutes. In those patients who are not converted to normal sinus rhythm, the drug will very often at least slow the ventricular response, making the patient more comfortable and allowing the blood pressure to increase.

Verapamil appears to work by prolonging the effective refractory period in cardiac tissues, and specifically by slowing the rate of firing in the sinoatrial (SA) node and slowing the rate of conduction in the atrioventricular (AV) node. Its major toxic effects include causing vasodilatation (with resultant hypotension), causing severe AV block, and causing sinus arrest.

Although verapamil is probably the best drug to use in this situation (having proven itself superior to propranolol and digoxin in this instance), remember that there are several simple maneuvers that can also convert the arrhythmia to normal sinus rhythm. If you can increase the patient's vagal tone (by massaging her carotid sinus or dunking her face in ice water) and thereby increase the vagal effects on both the sinoatrial and atrioventricular nodes, then the patient may well convert to normal sinus rhythm even without drug therapy. Although actual studies are few and far between, it appears that such maneuvers can be successful in a significant subset of such patients.

drug over the next 3 months to prevent new clots from forming, which drug would you pick?

2. Several weeks later, you see another patient recovering from surgery who has a red, swollen, and painful leg like the first patient. However, he suddenly complains of sharp pleuritic pain, coughs up a small amount of blood, becomes tachycardic and short of breath, and passes out. You measure his blood pressure, and find that it has suddenly dropped from 120/80 mm Hg to 60/30 mm Hg. What do you think happened? If you are correct, what would be your acute therapeutic goals? How would you achieve them?

ANSWERS

1. In this type of stable patient, you are not primarily concerned with rapidly lysing the clot already present. Rather, you simply want to prevent new clots from forming in the leg and embolizing to the lungs. Natural fibrinolysis will occur over days to weeks, and gradually "dissolve" or recanalize much of the clot. On the other hand, you would like to choose an anticoagulant that would work promptly to keep new clots from forming.

The drug of choice for prophylaxis against thrombosis or further clot formation during and following surgery is heparin. Its anticoagulant effect (partially mediated by its ability to activate antithrombin III) is immediate following intravenous injection. Although heparin has a rapid onset, it has the disadvantage that it must be given parenterally.

Once the situation is under control, you will want to start the patient on an oral anticoagulant such as warfarin. The effects of warfarin are slow to develop because it interferes with the synthesis of vitamin K–dependent clotting factors (II, VII, IX, X) by the liver, and several days may be required to deplete the blood of preformed clotting factors. During that 4 to 6 day period, you will want to continue the heparin infusion. Thus warfarin has the disadvantage of slow onset of action, but the advantage of ease of outpatient, oral administration.

2. It is likely that this patient has experienced a massive acute pulmonary embolism with significant obstruction of the pulmonary arteries. Documented massive pulmonary embolism with shock is a medical emergency, and several studies suggest that prompt treatment with agents that can dissolve or lyse the thromboemboli can result in more rapid improvement in a number of physiologic parameters. Anticoagulants such as warfarin or heparin can only prevent new clots from forming, but they cannot help dissolve the clot already present.

Clot lysis can be achieved by injecting streptokinase in patients who have not previously received the drug, or urokinase if it is suspected that the patient may be allergic to streptokinase. Both drugs act (in slightly different ways) to activate plasminogen, the body's intrinsic lytic agent. By activating plasminogen to plasmin, fibrinolysis is enhanced, and the blood clots in the leg and the pulmonary circulation will dissolve more quickly. If 24 hours of fibrinolytic therapy is successful, the patient will still need to go on to a course of heparin, and then a course of oral warfarin.

Treatment with sequential streptokinase/heparin causes more bleeding problems than treatment with heparin alone. Therefore, before initiating treatment with a fibrinolytic agent, it is very important to firmly establish the diagnosis, and to carefully consider the absolute and relative contraindications to the use of these agents (e.g., recent surgery, trauma, CPR). The potential benefits and potential risks vary with each individual patient.

SECTION EIGHT

CHEMOTHERAPY

CHAPTER 51

ALKYLATING AGENTS AND ANTIMETABOLITES

Related Readings

Clark et al: Chapter 60, pp. 702-708
Craig and Stitzel: Chapter 59, pp. 797-813
Gilman et al: Chapter 55, pp. 1247-1280
Katzung: Chapter 58, pp. 665-678

Key Concepts

- Cyclophosphamide: actions and pharmacokinetics
- Methotrexate: actions and pharmacokinetics

QUESTIONS

1. Two women with breast cancer are given cyclophosphamide to control their metastatic disease. The women are similar with respect to age, weight, and liver function. However, the first patient has a creatinine clearance of 100 ml/minute, and is receiving probenecid to treat her hyperuricemia and gout. The second woman has a creatinine clearance of 20 ml/minute. How does cyclophosphamide work? Do you anticipate different responses to the drug in the two patients?

2. The same two women return later for treatment with methotrexate. How does this drug work? Do you anticipate different responses to the drug in the two patients?

ANSWERS

1. Cyclophosphamide is an alkylating agent of the nitrogen mustard type, but it is stable enough that it can be given by mouth. In the liver it is activated by mixed function oxidases to at least two cytotoxic metabolites that escape to the blood and find their way to the tumor. One of those forms reacts covalently with DNA to produce crosslinks between the strands. The cell then dies because of an inability to replicate its DNA. One or both of these cytotoxic forms probably is excreted into the urine, where it produces cystitis in up to 10% of all patients treated. Patients should be encouraged to drink ample amounts of fluids and to void frequently to prevent this adverse reaction.

One of the women has a normal creatinine clearance of 100 ml/minute. The other clearly has compromised renal function. The second patient with the creatinine clearance of only 20 ml/minute may be more likely to develop cystitis or to experience systemic toxicity from cyclophosphamide since she will be less able to clear the cytotoxic metabolites and may void less frequently.

As far as is known, probenecid does not interfere with either the hepatic clearance (metabolism) or renal clearance (elimination) of cyclophosphamide or its metabolites.

2. Methotrexate is an antimetabolite that inhibits the enzyme dihydrofolate reductase. Like folic acid, methotrexate binds to the enzyme. However, methotrexate binds much more tightly than does folic acid, and thereby competitively inhibits the reduction of folic acid to tetrahydrofolate (Fig 51-1). As a consequence of this inhibition, there are diminished cellular levels of reduced folates, which are essential in one-carbon transfer reactions necessary for the synthesis of purines and some pyrimidines. Thus, methotrexate's cytotoxic effects are relatively specific for the S-phase of the cell cycle.

Since it is an analog of folic acid, methotrexate is itself a weak acid, and it is actively secreted by the renal tubule. Probenecid is also a weak acid that is secreted by the same mechanism. In the presence of probenecid the clearance of many organic acid drugs, including methotrexate, will be decreased, and the terminal slow phase of methotrexate elimination will be prolonged. Prolonged serum levels of methotrexate may result in greater ef-

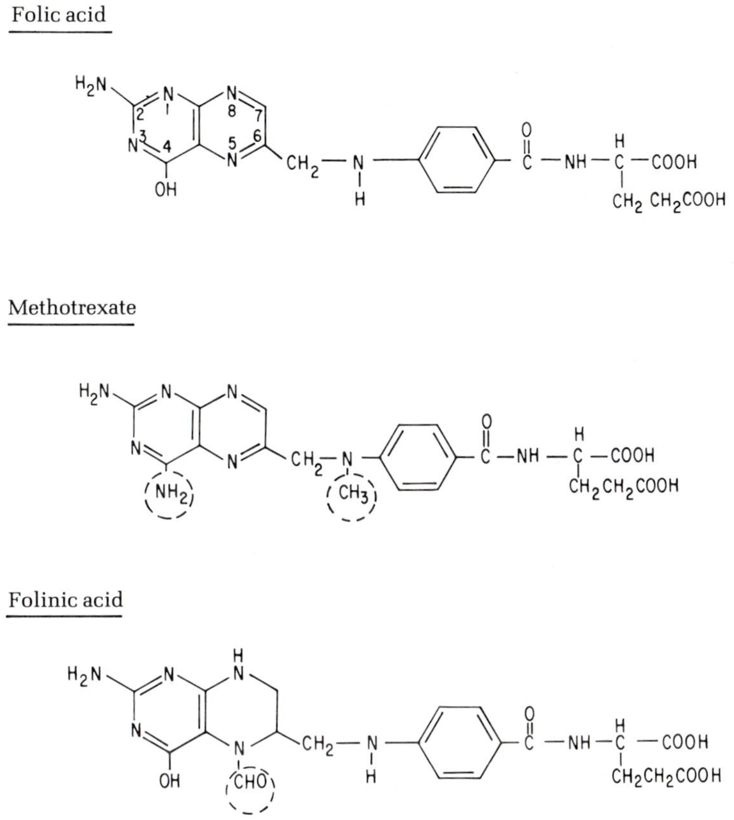

FIG. 51-1. Structures of folic acid, methotrexate, and folinic acid. Note that folinic acid is an "antidote" for methotrexate, since it is both a tetrahydrofolate (reduced at positions 5,6,7, and 8), and carries a formyl group (attached to N5) that can be used in one-carbon transfer reactions.

ficacy, but they also frequently result in more serious toxicity—renal toxicity, bone marrow suppression, and mucositis.

The second patient has compromised renal function with a creatinine clearance of only 20 ml/minute. Since renal dysfunction will likewise slow the excretion of methotrexate, this patient will likely encounter increased toxicity if she receives a standard dose. In fact, both the presence of renal dysfunction and the co-administration of probenecid are strong relative contraindications to the use of methotrexate.

CHAPTER 52

ANTINEOPLASTIC ANTIBIOTICS

Related Readings

Clark et al: Chapter 60, pp. 709-711
Craig and Stitzel: Chapter 58, pp. 813-819
Gilman et al: Chapter 55, pp. 1281-1289
Katzung: Chapter 58, pp. 678-682

Key Concepts

- Doxorubicin: actions, pharmacokinetics, and adverse effects
- Bleomycin: actions, pharmacokinetics, and adverse effects

QUESTIONS

1. Doxorubicin (Adriamycin™) is one of the most clinically useful anticancer antibiotics. It is active against many solid tumors and leukemias. How does this drug work?

A patient with a pancreatic tumor obstructing the common bile duct and resultant liver dysfunction receives this drug as part of an experimental protocol. What would happen to the drug's pattern of elimination and to drug toxicity?

2. A patient received combination chemotherapy directed against a testicular tumor. One of the drugs used was bleomycin. Why would this drug be a useful component of a combination regimen?

Several months into treatment, the patient began to complain of increasing shortness of breath, even though he had no previous history of any pulmonary disease. There is no evidence of pulmonary infection. What would concern you?

ANSWERS

1. Doxorubicin probably exerts its antineoplastic effects by several biochemical mechanisms. It can intercalate with DNA to interfere with its ability to direct DNA and RNA synthesis. Doxorubicin also produces single-stranded and double-stranded breaks in DNA as well as sister chromatid exchange. The strand breaks probably occur by a free radical mechanism, in which a semiquinone metabolite of doxorubicin generated by cytochrome P450 in the liver reacts with molecular oxygen to produce superoxide anions. The superoxide anions initiate free radical "showers" that are highly destructive to cells.

Doxorubicin is conjugated in the liver and the products are excreted in the bile. It has a very high hepatic clearance, amounting to 60% of liver blood flow. Severe toxicity may occur in patients with impaired liver function (e.g., obstruction of the common bile duct); with reduced hepatic clearance, elimination of the drug will be delayed. The most serious toxicities include bone marrow suppression and a cardiomyopathy.

2. Bleomycin is a good candidate for combination chemotherapy in this situation because it exhibits good activity against this type of tumor, and it has minimal bone marrow and immunosuppressive activity. The majority of other cancer chemotherapeutic agents have those kinds of effects that are dose-limiting with respect to their use. For example, if bleomycin is used in combination with an alkylating agent its therapeutic effects may be additive or even greater than additive to those of the alkylating agent, but the toxic effects will not overlap, so that each can be used in maximal doses.

Unfortunately, this particular patient appears to have fallen victim to an unusual but well-described toxic effect of bleomycin, namely damage to the lungs (interstitial pneumonitis) that can progress to pulmonary fibrosis. This effect of bleomycin also appears to be mediated by the generation of free radicals, since oxygen makes the reaction more severe. If appropriate tests confirm this adverse drug reaction, then the drug must be stopped at once to avoid serious or even fatal pulmonary damage.

CHAPTER 53

IMMUNOSUPPRESSIVE DRUGS

Related Readings

Clark et al: Chapter 61
Craig and Stitzel: Chapter 60
Gilman et al: Chapter 55, pp. 1276-1277 and 1298-1299
Katzung: Chapter 59

Key Concepts

- Azathioprine: actions, pharmacokinetics, and interaction with allopurinol
- Cyclosporine: actions, indications, and adverse effects

QUESTIONS

1. A patient with vasculitis has the condition well controlled with a stable daily dose of Imuran™. What is Imuran™? How does it work? After 3 months, a new intern notices that the patient has asymptomatic hyperuricemia, and prescribes Zyloprim™. What is that drug, and how does it work? What do you think will happen to the patient?

2. Cyclosporine is one of our newest and most exciting immunosuppressive agents. Its availability may allow us to use much lower doses of toxic drugs, such as azathioprine and prednisone. Without this drug, heart and liver transplantation would probably not be possible. How does the drug work? What is its most common indication? Do you see any problems with its use in that situation?

ANSWERS

1. Imuran™ is the trade name for azathioprine, a prodrug that is metabolized to form the immunosuppressive agent, 6-mercaptopurine (6-MP), a purine antimetabolite (Fig. 53-1). Although it is still not entirely clear how 6-MP produces its immunosuppressive effects, it appears that 6-MP is metabolized to the ribonucleotide, 6-thioinosine-5′-phosphate (6-thioIMP). This ribonucleotide may go on to inhibit several vital metabolic reactions. 6-MP is ultimately metabolized by xanthine oxidase, first to 6-thioxanthine, then to 6-thiouric acid (Fig. 53-1). Zyloprim™ is the trade name for allopurinol, an inhibitor of xanthine oxidase used in patients with recurrent gout or hyperuricemia who overproduce uric acid. As mentioned above, 6-MP is also metabolized by the enzyme, xanthine oxidase. Indeed, allopurinol was originally developed to prolong the biologic half-life of 6-MP to make it a more effective antineoplastic agent. If allopurinol is used in combination with azathioprine, it will also prolong the half-life of 6-MP and intensify its toxic effects. The dosage of azathioprine should be reduced to one-fourth the usual dosage in that circumstance to avoid toxicity.

2. Cyclosporine is a recently developed peptide antibiotic with immunosuppresive properties. Although its precise mechanism of action is not known, it may inhibit the production of T-cell growth factors. It may do this by inhibiting lymphokine (interleukin-2) production by activated T-helper cells, by blocking the acquisition of receptors for interleukin-2 by precursor cytotoxic T-cells, or by decreasing the responsiveness of helper/inducer T-cells to interleukin-1.

Its most common indication is in allogeneic organ transplants such as kidney, liver, heart, heart-lung, or pancreas to prevent rejection by the host. Since kidney transplants are presently the most common type of organ transplant procedure, the drug's most common indication is to prevent rejection of a kidney allograft. It may be used by itself, or with low doses of other immunosuppressive agents such as prednisone or azathioprine.

Some of the drug's adverse effects include nephrotoxicity, liver dysfunction, and increased infections, but little bone marrow suppression. After patients have received their kidney transplants, a deterioration in renal function may be difficult to evaluate. If the deterioration represents graft rejec-

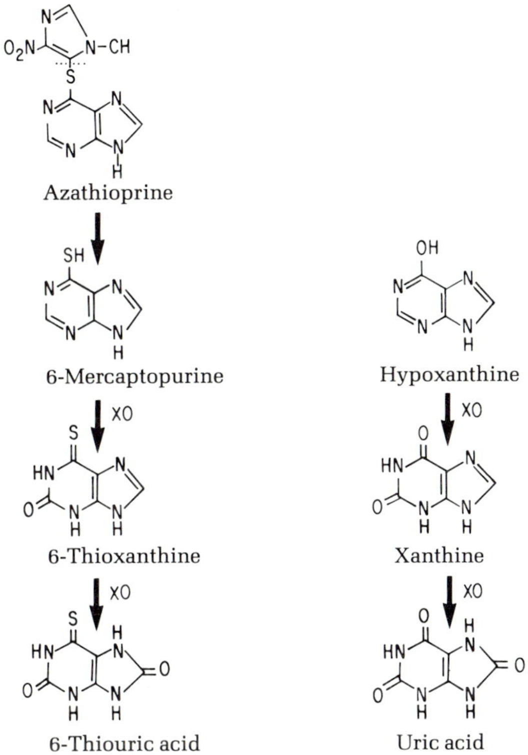

FIG. 53-1. Structure and metabolism of azathioprine. Azathioprine is cleaved to form 6-mercaptopurine (6-MP), which is then metabolized by the enzyme xanthine oxidase (X.O.) to form 6-thioxanthine and 6-thiouric acid. The structures of hypoxanthine, xanthine, and uric acid are also shown for the sake of comparison.

tion, then more cyclosporine may be useful. If the deterioration represents cyclosporine nephrotoxicity, then a lower dose may be indicated. As you can see, the use of cyclosporine in patients with kidney transplants has been extremely useful, but interpretation and treatment of increasing renal dysfunction after transplantation has become more challenging.

CHAPTER 54

ANTIVIRAL AND ANTIFUNGAL DRUGS

Related Readings

Clark et al: Chapter 54; Chapter 55, pp. 679-681
Craig and Stitzel: Chapters 52 and 56
Gilman et al: Chapter 54
Katzung: Chapters 48 and 49

Key Concepts

- Azidothymidine: mechanism of action and adverse effects
- Amphotericin B: mechanism of action and adverse effects

QUESTIONS

1. One of the most promising antiviral drugs that seems to benefit some patients with symptomatic human immunodeficiency virus (HIV) infections is the drug known as AZT. What is this drug, and how does it work? What is the major side effect that has forced many such patients to discontinue taking the drug?

2. A debilitated cancer patient has bone marrow that is just beginning to recover from previous chemotherapy. He is still receiving three antibiotics to treat a presumed (but never proven) bacterial infection. An alert intern notices several new small pustules; a properly stained specimen of the pus reveals a yeast infection. At the same time, a blood culture grows out *Candida albicans*. Just before going off duty, the intern orders a new drug to treat the fungemia. The patient receives the first dose intravenously, and immediately develops shortness of breath, hives, hypotension, fever, and shaking. You are called to see the patient. What do you think might be going on?

ANSWERS

1. Azidothymidine (AZT, azidodideoxythymidine) is an antiviral agent that is an analog (antimetabolite) of deoxythymidine (Fig. 54-1). It appears to act primarily by inhibiting viral reverse transcriptase to block the synthesis of DNA from the viral RNA template. It is of considerable current interest because it has demonstrated some beneficial effects (prolongation of survival, fewer symptoms) in some specific groups of patients with AIDS and AIDS-related syndromes.

There is concern about extrapolating these exciting preliminary results prematurely to all patients with AIDS or all patients infected with HIV. One important limiting factor of AZT is a late-occurring severe anemia caused

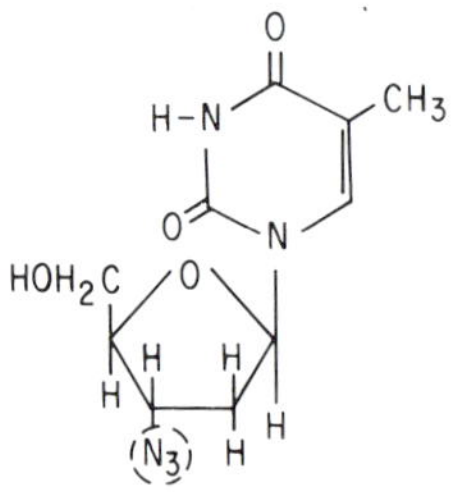

Azidothymidine

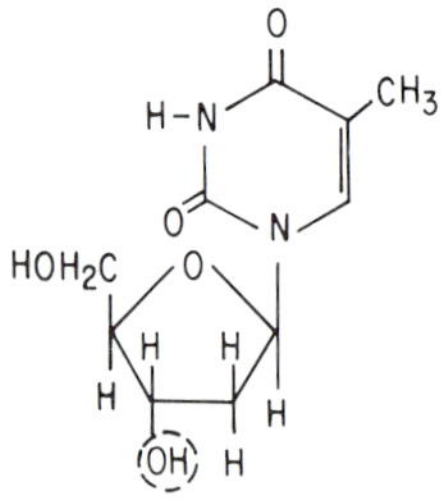

Thymidine

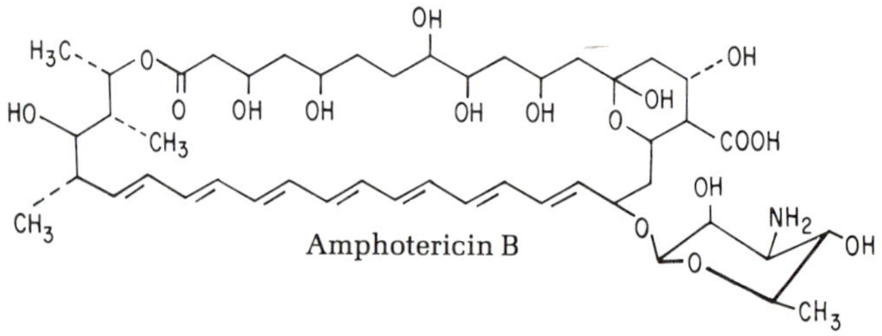

Amphotericin B

FIG. 54-1. Structures of azidothymidine (azidodideoxythymidine), thymidine (deoxythymidine), and amphotericin B.

by bone marrow depression. Given this potentially severe toxic effect, the extrapolation of preliminary exciting results found in specific small groups of patients to much larger groups of patients—without firm scientific data—has proven to be problematic and controversial.

2. The drug given was most likely amphotericin B, which has good activity against many *Candida* species including *albicans*. The drug contains a large ring structure and many double bonds, and is very poorly soluble in water (Fig. 54-1). It appears to bind tightly to the fungal cell membrane, and thereby alters the membrane's permeability and transport properties. Perhaps half of all patients receiving the drug intravenously for the first time develop fever, chills, and vomiting. These symptoms, although worrisome, can often be reduced or prevented by giving a smaller dose, by premedicating the patient with appropriate drugs (e.g., corticosteroids, antihistamines), or by treating the symptoms (e.g., acetaminophen for fever, meperidine for rigors).

More ominous in this patient are the associated symptoms of shortness of breath, hives, and hypotension. These symptoms indicate the presence of a more severe adverse reaction, perhaps even an anaphylactoid reaction (similar to an anaphylactic reaction, but without evidence of an immunologic basis). The amphotericin should be stopped immediately, and you should be prepared to administer epinephrine and other second-line drugs.

CHAPTER 55

PENICILLIN

Related Readings

Clark et al: Chapter 53, pp. 642-651
Craig and Stitzel: Chapter 47, pp. 654-673
Gilman et al: Chapter 50, pp. 1115-1137
Katzung: Chapter 43, pp. 516-522

Key Concepts

- Properties of aqueous crystalline penicillin G
- Properties of procaine penicillin G
- Properties of benzathine penicillin G
- Properties of oral penicillin G

QUESTIONS

1. A 63-year-old man develops acute pneumococcal pneumonia complicated by pneumococcal meningitis. This is a life-threatening infection in which the bacteria have entered the bloodstream (bacteremia) from the infection in the lungs, and spread via the bloodstream to the meninges and cerebrospinal fluid. High serum levels of penicillin G must be achieved, so that the lower levels found in the cerebrospinal fluid are still bactericidal. What penicillin preparation would be best in this situation?

2. A 37-year-old man with urethral gonorrhea lives in a locality that has not experienced significant resistance of the organism to penicillin. What penicillin preparation is most often used to treat this disease?

3. A 9-year-old girl recovering from acute rheumatic fever requires continuous prophylaxis for at least several years to protect her damaged mitral valve. She is unreliable when it comes to taking pills. What type of penicillin preparation would be most useful in preventing recurrent streptococcal infection and recurrent rheumatic fever?

4. A 24-year-old medical student develops mild pneumococcal pneumonia. He is reliable, is having no difficulty eating or drinking, and desires to be treated on an outpatient basis because of exams. What type of penicillin preparation would be easiest for him to take as an outpatient?

ANSWERS

1. *Streptococcus pneumoniae (Pneumococcus)* is almost always sensitive to penicillin G, which is the drug of choice in this infection. Penicillin G (benzylpenicillin) is the simplest of the penicillins, and closely related to 6-aminopenicillanic acid, the parent compound (Fig. 55-1). Other penicillin derivatives are also related to this parent compound. If the infection were a simple pneumonia, or even a pneumonia with associated bacteremia, smaller doses of penicillin could be used because the organism is so sensitive. However, very high penicillin levels in serum must be attained for drug levels in the spinal fluid (which are often 10% or less of the serum concentration) to be effective. These high serum penicillin levels can best be attained by giving large doses of penicillin G intravenously.

The only pharmaceutical preparation of penicillin G that is designed to be given intravenously is the crystalline form of penicillin G, which is available as either a sodium or potassium salt, and is given as an aqueous solution. Since the elimination half-life of penicillin G is only about ½ hour, we usually give a dose (2 million units) intravenously every 2 hours. Under these conditions penicillin has reduced the death rate from pneumo-

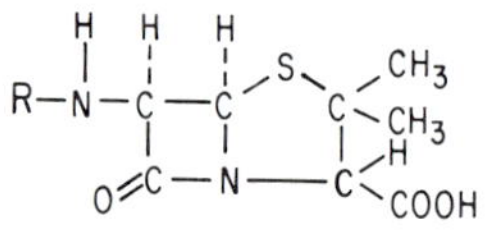

Substituted 6-aminopenicillanic acid

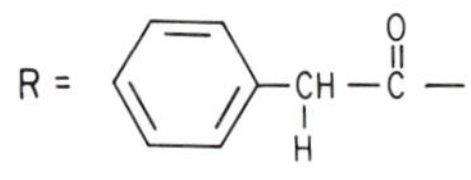

Penicillin G

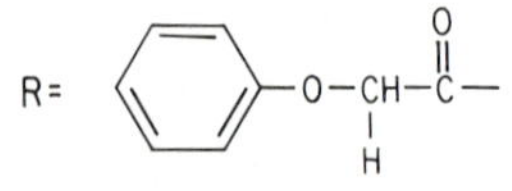

Penicillin V

FIG. 55-1. Structures of 6-aminopenicillanic acid, penicillin G (benzylpenicillin), and penicillin V (phenoxymethylpenicillin).

coccal meningitis from almost 100% to between 8% and 25%. You can see that penicillin has earned its reputation as a wonder drug.

2. It is highly desirable to provide a curative dose of antibiotic at the time of diagnosis, because gonococcal disease is primarily sexually transmitted and infected patients may not comply with lengthy oral treatment plans. Fortunately, the pathogen in this disease (a species of *Neisseria*) is usually quite sensitive to penicillin G. However, moderate serum levels of penicillin G must be maintained for up to 24 hours to have a high chance of curing the infection.

Fortunately, there is a pharmaceutical preparation of penicillin G that provides such a drug profile. Penicillin G procaine suspension is a preparation with only moderate water solubility. Because of its intermediate rate of absorption after intramuscular (IM) injection, it achieves moderate serum concentrations that persist for up to 24 hours. This patient could be managed with procaine penicillin G suspension 4.8 million units intramuscularly, which can be given during the initial visit to the clinic.

Cure rates can be improved by causing a deliberate drug interaction. Penicillin is eliminated almost entirely by the kidney via active tubular secretion. This weak organic acid transport system is markedly inhibited by the drug, probenecid. Therefore, probenecid 1 g taken orally is usually given before the intramuscular injection of penicillin G procaine suspension to slow the renal elimination of the absorbed penicillin G.

3. Prevention of future streptococcal infections requires very low serum concentrations of penicillin G—much lower levels than are needed in the treatment of such diseases. However, these low serum levels must be maintained for months or even years. Unfortunately, this patient would almost certainly miss many doses if oral penicillin (to be taken four times daily) were prescribed.

In this case, it would be advantageous to have a repository form of penicillin G available, which could be given intramuscularly perhaps once each month to provide a low but sustained serum level of penicillin. Fortunately, still another pharmaceutical formulation of penicillin G is available with just these properties.

Penicillin G benzathine suspension is even less water-soluble than the procaine suspension described above. After it has been intramuscularly injected, it is very slowly absorbed over periods up to 1 month, yielding quite low but sustained serum levels of penicillin G. Although such low serum levels would be inadequate in the treatment of serious pneumococcal disease or gonorrhea, these levels are ideal for the prevention (prophylaxis) of future streptococcal disease, including rheumatic fever.

4. Obviously, the most convenient form of penicillin for this student to take as an outpatient would be tablets of penicillin G. Oral penicillin G usually achieves sufficiently high serum concentrations to kill the very sensitive *Pneumococcus* organisms. However, penicillin G is not very resistant to the destructive effects of the acidic environment of the stomach. Penicillin V (phenoxymethylpenicillin, Fig. 55-1) has a similar effect on *Pneumococcus* as penicillin G, but it is much more resistant to the acid pH of the stomach. Thus, if a course of oral penicillin were given in this case, penicillin V would be the optimal drug.

• • •

As you can see, penicillin G is a fascinating drug. Actually, it is really a group of pharmaceutical preparations with very different properties and indications. Before prescribing penicillin G, you must decide what type of pharmacokinetic profile you desire, and then order the appropriate pharmaceutical preparation to provide the desired characteristics of serum concentration, duration of effect, route of administration, rate of absorption, and resistance to gastric pH.

CHAPTER 56

PENICILLIN DERIVATIVES

Related Readings

Clark et al: Chapter 53, pp. 642-651
Craig and Stitzel: Chapter 47, pp. 654-673
Gilman et al: Chapter 50, pp. 1115-1137
Katzung: Chapter 43, pp. 516-522

Key Concepts

- Properties of ampicillin
- Properties of mezlocillin
- Properties of nafcillin and dicloxacillin

QUESTIONS

1. A 24-year-old female medical student develops acute cystitis. There is no evidence of systemic illness or pyelonephritis. She feels well otherwise, with no fever, rigors, nausea, or vomiting. Could you use a penicillin derivative to treat her infection?

2. A hospitalized 65-year-old diabetic woman develops pyuria while her Foley catheter is in place. A sample of urine is sent to the laboratory to be cultured, and the bladder catheter is removed. The next night, she develops what appears to be a classic case of sepsis, with high fever, rigors, nausea, vomiting, and mild hypotension. The only source for her sepsis seems to be her cloudy urine, which the laboratory reports is growing greater than 100,000 *E. coli* sensitive to ampicillin. How would you treat this patient?

3. A 45-year-old man develops a large carbuncle on his neck; he treats it himself with pushing, poking, and hot soaks. It gradually resolves after several weeks of being red, swollen, tender, hot, and draining pus. He is admitted to the hospital after he develops shaking chills, fever, muscle aches, backache, shortness of breath, and a new murmur of mild aortic regurgitation. What do you think is going on? How would you treat the patient initially? After 4 weeks in the hospital, the patient insists on leaving the hospital. Could you continue treatment?

4. A 42-year-old man is being treated for acute myelogenous leukemia. During his period of drug-induced pancytopenia he develops pneumonia, and laboratory tests reveal gram-negative rods. He appears septic as well (fever, chills, mild hypotension). What types of antibiotics would be useful here?

ANSWERS

1. The most common organism involved in uncomplicated urinary tract infections in women is *E. coli*. This organism, when acquired in the community, is usually sensitive to a variety of antibiotics, including the penicillin derivative ampicillin (Fig. 56-1). Ampicillin is similar to penicillin G in many ways, but it has increased activity against many common gram-negative rods and has good oral bioavailability. Since ampicillin is concentrated in the urine and since this patient could easily take oral medications, her mild bladder infection could be treated with a course of oral ampicillin. Because it concentrates in the urine and it has a wide spectrum of activity, ampicillin is also a useful drug in men with urinary tract infections caused by gram-positive cocci as well.

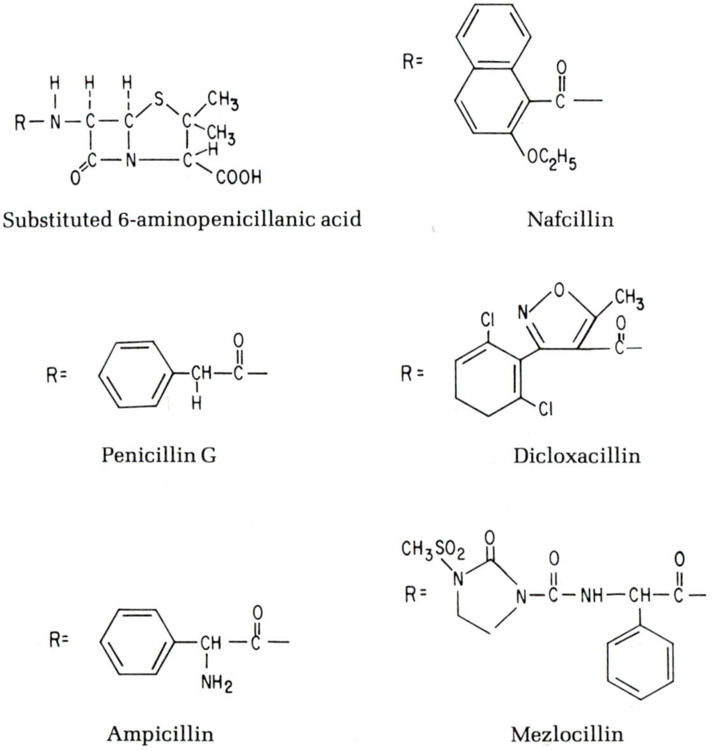

FIG. 56-1. Structures of penicillin G, ampicillin, nafcillin, dicloxacillin, and mezlocillin.

2. Like the first patient, this woman also has a bladder infection caused by *E. coli*. However, her cystitis (bladder infection) appears to have progressed to cause pyelonephritis and urosepsis as well, possibly because of her underlying diabetes. Although urinary tract infections acquired in the hospital can be caused by a variety of bacteria and are often resistant to ampicillin, fortunately in this case the earlier urine culture confirmed that the pathogen was indeed a species of *E. coli* sensitive to ampicillin.

However, since this woman is more seriously ill and possibly has bacteremia, much higher serum concentrations of ampicillin are required than in the previous case. In addition, because of her nausea and vomiting, this patient cannot take oral medications. For both of these reasons, an intravenous preparation of ampicillin should be used to treat this life-threatening infection.

3. Most carbuncles, such as the one described in this case, are caused by *Staphylococcus aureus*. This unpleasant local infection sounds like it is starting to improve. However, the new symptoms strongly suggest that the patient has developed a new case of septicemia, and possibly bacteremia as well. The most likely cause would be that while the patient was poking his carbuncle, he caused a transient episode of bacteremia to occur. These staphylococci lodged on his aortic valve and began to grow, causing an acute case of staphylococcal endocarditis (infection of a heart valve). This is an extremely serious infection in any patient; in this patient, the development of a new murmur of aortic regurgitation is a grave prognostic sign. Blood samples must be cultured to confirm the diagnosis, and treatment must be started immediately with a drug that will kill the most likely pathogen. Thus, a drug is required that can achieve high concentrations in plasma, and that will be resistant to the beta-lactamases (penicillinases) produced by most strains of *Staphylococcus aureus*.

The best drug in this situation is a large intravenous dose of nafcillin, another penicillin derivative (Fig. 56-1). Nafcillin belongs to a group of penicillin derivatives (including methicillin and oxacillin) that were specially designed for their anti-staphylococcal properties. Although they are less effective against gram-negative rods, they demonstrate superb activity against most staphylococci.

Such severe bacteremias, when resulting from endocarditis, should be treated for 6 weeks. We used to insist on 6 weeks of treatment with intravenous nafcillin. However, some recent studies have suggested that the last 2 to 3 weeks of therapy can be accomplished with oral drugs, as long as those drugs have excellent oral bioavailability and good anti-staphylococcal coverage. The best such drug is dicloxacillin (Fig. 56-1). Dicloxacillin is similar in coverage to nafcillin, but it is specifically formulated for oral administration. Thus, for selected patients, part of the long course of antibiotic therapy can be accomplished as an outpatient, with oral medications.

4. When such patients receive chemotherapy to treat their leukemias, they often develop severe bone marrow depression, resulting in a severe drop in their white blood cell counts. During this period of neutropenia, they often become infected and exhibit signs of sepsis. When such patients develop signs of pneumonia and sepsis, the pathogen very often originates from the patient's own gastrointestinal tract, usually a gram-negative rod, as was found in this case.

Since the patient is so ill, and since the exact identity and sensitivity of the gram-negative rod is not known, many experts recommend beginning treatment with two antibiotics, both active against the types of gram-negative rods often found in such cases. Important pathogens include *E. coli*, *Enterobacter* sp., and *Pseudomonas aeruginosa*.

Another family of penicillin derivatives has been synthesized and gives an extremely good spectrum of activity against many of these gram-negative rods, including *Pseudomonas aeruginosa*. This group includes mezlocillin, carbenicillin, ticarcillin, piperacillin, and azlocillin. The structure of a commonly-used member of this group, mezlocillin, is also seen in Fig. 56-1.

As you can see from these questions, penicillin derivatives have come to play an extremely important role in the treatment of bacterial infections. No one drug or class seems to be "best" against all pathogens. Rather, each group of penicillin derivatives has relative strengths and weaknesses, and should be used only in appropriate situations.

CHAPTER 57

MECHANISMS OF DRUG RESISTANCE

Related Readings

Clark et al: Chapter 51 and Chapter 60
Craig and Stitzel: Chapter 45 and Chapter 59, pp. 806-809
Gilman et al: Chapter 48 and Chapter 55, pp. 1263-1267
Katzung: Chapter 42 and Chapter 58, pp. 674-675

Key Concepts

- Mechanisms of development of cancer cell resistance to methotrexate
- Mechanisms of development of bacterial resistance to antibiotics

QUESTIONS

1. One of the major problems for oncologists is that tumor cells may become resistant to antineoplastic drugs. For example, a patient may have a tumor that is initially responsive to methotrexate: the first few doses cause the tumor to shrink dramatically, perhaps even to the point where there is no evident or measurable disease (a remission). However, the tumor may recur several months later, and when treatment with methotrexate is again attempted, there is no obvious response. What possible mechanisms of tumor cell resistance to methotrexate could have developed?

2. A new aminoglycoside antibiotic is introduced into your hospital formulary. Its use by doctors is not controlled, and many patients receive this antibiotic, even when older antibiotics such as ampicillin would work just as well. At first, more than 99% of the gram-negative rods isolated in the hospital microbiology laboratory are sensitive to this new antibiotic. Over the next 12 months, however, several of the more invasive strains of gram-negative rods became increasingly resistant to the antibiotic. In some strains, such as *Pseudomonas* species, almost 50% of the isolates have become resistant to this new antibiotic. How have these resistant strains of bacteria "learned" to become resistant?

ANSWERS

1. Cancer cells may rapidly develop resistance to the cytotoxic effects of methotrexate, thus causing a significant problem for oncologists who are trying to control a neoplastic disease. Several biochemical mechanisms are responsible for this development of resistance. One mechanism of resistance involves an impairment of the transport of methotrexate into the cancer cells. The drug must penetrate the cell membrane to be effective.

Another mechanism is that the cancer cells begin to make isoenzymes of dihydrofolate reductase that have a decreased affinity for methotrexate. The cytotoxic activity of methotrexate depends on its great affinity for this enzyme and its ability to bind to (and thus inhibit) the enzyme when present at low concentrations. If the affinity of the enzyme for the drug is decreased, the cytotoxic activity is also decreased.

Finally, the synthesis of normal dihydrofolate reductase seems to be induced by treatment with the drug. Through gene amplification of the DNA coding for this enzyme, increased mRNA and increased enzyme itself are synthesized. If more enzyme is available, standard concentrations of methotrexate will obviously be less effective.

Thus, cancer cells have demonstrated at least three distinct mechanisms for acquiring resistance to this antineoplastic agent. It is likely that additional mechanisms of drug resistance will be found responsible for similar problems occurring with other antineoplastic agents.

2. Bacteria can acquire resistance to aminoglycoside antibiotics by several biochemical mechanisms. Clinically, the most important mechanism appears to be that the bacteria synthesize enzymes for deactivating the antibiotics by phosphorylating, adenylating, or acetylating critical and specific amino or hydroxyl groups on the drugs. This type of resistance is usually coded for on plasmids, which has important implications for the spreading of resistance from one strain to another.

The bacterial ribosome may change in such a way that the affinity of the aminoglycoside for it is lowered, which decreases the drug's antibacterial activity. This change in the ribosomal protein may occur as a result of chromosomal mutation.

Finally, the cell surface of the bacteria may change in such a way that the drug fails to permeate (or be transported into) the outer membrane of gram-negative organisms. These alterations in the cell surface can be coded for in the bacterial genome or in plasmids.

Unfortunately, when resistance develops to one antibiotic, the bacterium may simultaneously develop resistance to other antibiotics as well. Antibiotic therapy is a two-edged sword, and treatment must be designed in such a way as to maximize the benefits for the patient and minimize the chance of promoting increased bacterial resistance.

SECTION NINE

TOXICOLOGY

CHAPTER 58

HEAVY METALS AND CHELATORS

Related Readings

Clark et al: Chapter 62
Craig and Stitzel: Chapter 8, pp. 120-123
Gilman et al: Chapter 69
Katzung: Chapter 61

Key Concepts

- Symptoms and treatment of chronic lead toxicity
- Symptoms and treatment of acute iron poisoning

QUESTIONS

1. A 55-year-old iron salvage worker began a new job 3 months ago. He and his partner were responsible for dismantling a 65-year-old steel bridge that had originally been painted a dull red color. With acetylene torches they gradually broke up the entire structure of the bridge, and reduced it to small pieces of junk steel that could be removed.

After 2 months on the job, the worker began to experience continuous fatigue, weakness in the arms and legs, and loss of appetite. He also noted intermittent cramping abdominal pain, inability to concentrate, aching in both lower legs, and the unusual symptom of having the area around his mouth turn white. Evaluation revealed mild muscle weakness, a peripheral motor neuropathy, and a mild anemia with basophilic stippling of the red blood cells. What do you think caused this syndrome? How would you treat the patient?

2. An 18-month-old toddler was able to open a bottle of his mother's medication. When she found him, he had apparently ingested about 40 hydrated ferrous sulfate tablets (320 mg each). He appeared to be awake and alert, and quite proud of what he had accomplished. Needless to say, the mother was concerned and called the Regional Poison Control Center for advice. What do you think they suggested? What to you think was ultimately done?

ANSWERS

1. In a situation of this type, where metals are exposed to extreme temperatures (e.g., acetylene torches), it is often very difficult to assign responsibility for the appearance of toxic signs and symptoms to a particular agent. For example, the steel might have contained small amounts of cadmium, zinc, mercury, or copper. The inhalation of fumes of any of these could produce toxic signs, but the initial picture is usually that of respiratory tract involvement. In this case, the absence of respiratory tract involvement, the fact that the structure had been painted many times with a red pigmented paint, and the many clues provided by the systemic signs and symptoms suggest the diagnosis of chronic lead intoxication.

It would be appropriate to request a laboratory screening for heavy metals with particular attention being paid to blood lead levels. Lead-poisoned patients often exhibit colic, constipation, pallor, and muscle weakness. The first three signs are the result of spasmogenic effects of lead on visceral and vascular smooth muscle, and the last is caused by a poorly defined effect of lead on transmission at the myoneural junction. Anemia and basophilic stippling of red cells are also consistent with lead poisoning. If the laboratory workup reveals high levels of lead in the blood or urine, it would be appropriate to proceed with chelation therapy in an attempt to reduce the body's total burden of lead to nonsymptomatic levels.

The agent of choice for chronic lead poisoning without the complication of encephalopathy would be the calcium disodium ethylenediaminetetraacetic acid (EDTA) either by intravenous infusion or by repeated intramuscular injections. The blood levels should be evaluated after each course of therapy as well as the clinical response of the patient. Sometimes either dimercaprol (BAL) or D-penicillamine is also given in very severe cases or cases where the central nervous system involvement is extensive.

2. This is potentially a very serious intoxication. Severe poisoning and death have resulted in children after the ingestion of as few as 15 tablets of ferrous sulfate (320 mg of hydrated ferrous sulfate contains 64 mg elemental iron). Because this child currently appears to be in no distress, it is likely that the tablets were enteric coated. When these tablets pass from the stomach into the small intestine, the coating will dissolve and a fulminating poisoning will follow.

Every attempt should be made to remove the tablets as soon as possible before free ferrous sulfate is released to produce severe corrosive local lesions in the gastrointestinal tract or systemic poisoning from absorbed iron. The child should be given syrup of ipecac to induce vomiting, thus removing the intact tablets or unabsorbed ferrous sulfate. The alternative is gastric lavage, but a large bore tube must be used to remove undisintegrated tablets.

Once stomach evacuation has been accomplished, the physician should be prepared to administer deferoxamine to chelate the toxic levels of iron in the blood and hasten its urinary excretion. This chelating agent is considered to be an "antidote" for this specific intoxication. Measuring the serum iron level and the total iron binding capacity may be useful in helping to decide when to initiate chelation therapy. One should also be prepared to initiate measures for the management of shock and other possible complications of severe iron intoxication, including bloody diarrhea, coma, and hyperglycemia.

CHAPTER 59

SOLVENTS AND COMMERCIAL PRODUCTS

Related Readings

Clark et al: Chapter 62
Craig and Stitzel: Chapter 8
Gilman et al: Chapters 68 and 70
Katzung: Chapters 60 and 62

Key Concepts

- Toxicity and treatment of aliphatic hydrocarbon ingestion
- Toxicity and treatment of lye ingestion

QUESTIONS

1. A 42-year-old man owns a local nursery. One afternoon, he noted a slow leak of gasoline from the large fuel tank on one of his tractors. To prevent the gasoline from leaking into the ground, he decided to siphon the gas from the leaking tank into several 10 gallon gas tanks. He inserted a length of hose into the leaky tank, and primed the siphon by sucking on the distal end of the hose. The next thing he knew, his mouth was full of gasoline and he was overcome with a fit of coughing. The coughing and sense of gasoline on his breath persisted for about 30 minutes, and he was driven to a hospital. In the emergency room, his breath smelled like gasoline and he continued to cough. Examination of his lungs was normal, but his chest x-ray showed a consolidation of his right middle lobe. Arterial blood gases revealed very mild hypoxemia and hyperventilation. How would you treat this patient?

2. A 3-year-old child was playing in the kitchen one day and found a bottle of Drano™ under the kitchen sink. He drank several mouthfuls and then began shrieking. His mother found him crying hysterically, and took him immediately to the emergency room. On admission, he was crying and agitated, had burns about his lips and inside his mouth, and appeared to be drooling. He was given an injection of morphine for pain, and plans for management were discussed. How would you proceed in this situation?

ANSWERS

1. The clinical picture in this patient strongly suggests that he had aspirated gasoline (an aliphatic hydrocarbon mixture of appropriate viscosity to be dangerous) into his tracheobronchial tree. The respiratory signs and symptoms together with the chest x-ray indicate that an acute localized pneumonitis is developing, and it is potentially life-threatening if it progresses to diffuse involvement.

Aspiration has already occurred, so nothing can be done at this point to try to prevent it. You are now limited to providing good supportive and symptomatic care. There is probably little gasoline in the stomach, and thus the risks of evacuating the stomach (which might provoke another episode of gasoline pulmonary aspiration) outweigh the minimal benefits. If the patient becomes comatose, you could protect the airway from further insult and provide ventilatory assistance by putting a cuffed endotracheal tube in place. Respiratory function and pulmonary damage should be followed by serial lung examinations, chest x-rays, and arterial blood gases.

The patient should be put on a cardiac monitor. If arrhythmias occur (gasoline sensitizes the myocardium to adrenergic stimulation) intervention with antiarrhythmic drugs may be indicated. Antibiotics would be needed only if a bacterial pneumonitis intervenes.

2. The child should be given large volumes of water or milk if he can drink them. This will dilute the highly concentrated and corrosive alkali (sodium hydroxide) found in the drain cleaner. Whether or not one should attempt to neutralize the alkali in the stomach with such materials as orange juice or dilute vinegar (weak acids) is controversial. Gastric lavage or emetic drugs are contraindicated because of the danger of gastric or esophageal perforation. An injection of an appropriate dose of atropine may help suppress the hypersalivation.

Be prepared to treat shock by expanding the plasma or blood volume. Even if the patient survives the acute episode, there is the danger that he will develop a late esophageal perforation or stricture. Damage to the esophagus may be evaluated by fluoroscopy or endoscopy. If esophageal perforation and infection of the mediastinum develop, surgery and antibiotics will become necessary. If late strictures occur despite prophylactic measures, it may be necessary to resort to esophageal dilatation or reconstructive surgery.

As you can see, a small innocent-looking bottle of sodium hydroxide can produce a catastrophic, even fatal, ingestion.

CHAPTER 60

ASPHYXIANTS

Related Readings

Clark et al: Chapter 62
Craig and Stitzel: Chapter 8
Gilman et al: Chapter 70
Katzung: Chapter 60

Key Concepts

- Management of carbon monoxide poisoning
- Management of nitrogen dioxide poisoning

QUESTIONS

1. A 50-year-old police traffic officer had been hospitalized twice during the past 4 years with episodes of loss of consciousness.* Each episode occurred between 3 and 5 PM, with a feeling of lightheadedness for ½ to 2 hours duration, dizziness, ataxia, somnolence, and loss of consciousness for 15 to 90 minutes, during which his hands might twitch. There had been no tongue-biting or incontinence. He had undergone marked personality changes over the previous few months, becoming progressively more ner-

*This problem was simplified and adapted from a case previously reported. See Gilbert, GJ, and Glaser, GH: Neurologic manifestation of carbon monoxide poisoning, N. Eng. J. Med. 261:1217-1220, 1959.

vous, irritable, and unhappy. He had received phenytoin and phenobarbital for 2 years for presumed psychomotor epilepsy without any change in the "seizure" frequency. What else might account for his problem?

2. A 49-year-old firefighter was admitted with severe respiratory distress the day after he inhaled a toxic gas originating in a leak from a chemical plant.* He was exposed for only 10 minutes and initially experienced only a mild, transient headache and a dry, hacking cough. When he was admitted, he was cyanotic and febrile. His blood pressure was 140/100 mm Hg, his pulse was 136 BPM, and his respiratory rate was 44 breaths/minute. Auscultation of the lungs revealed diffuse rales and wheezes; the chest x-ray indicated pulmonary edema. The ECG suggested acute right ventricular strain. His condition deteriorated rapidly, and he was semicomatose within 30 minutes after he was admitted. What do you think he was exposed to, and how would you manage this patient?

*This problem was simplified and adapted from a case previously reported. See Tse, RL, and Bockman, AA: Nitrogen dioxide toxicity: report of four cases in firemen, JAMA 212:1341-1344, 1970.

ANSWERS

1. The absence of overt motor seizures, tongue-biting, and incontinence, together with a failure of antiepileptic therapy appropriate for psychomotor epilepsy would suggest that that diagnosis was incorrect. When seeking other causes, a number of clues can be found in the careful history that was taken. The individual was a traffic officer, and his problems always occurred at times associated with traffic rush hour. The clinical picture in combination with the history is consistent with a series of recurring acute intoxications with carbon monoxide.

Carbon monoxide has little or no tendency to produce persistent sequelae unless the exposure is so severe that the hypoxic insult leads to permanent nerve damage. In such cases, the sequelae are not specific for carbon monoxide, but may also result from asphyxia as a result of any cause (e.g., strangulation, near-drowning, or suffocation). Otherwise, full recovery is the general rule. If the patient had been brought in during an acute episode, a blood sample should have been drawn for a carboxyhemoglobin determination. The patient should receive 100% oxygen to breathe, to displace the carbon monoxide that is tightly bound to hemoglobin. If hyperbaric oxygen can be delivered (as in a pressure chamber), then the rate of displacement of carbon monoxide by oxygen will be even faster. After recovery, the patient should request reassignment to duty that reduces his risk of exposure to carbon monoxide.

2. Firefighters are often exposed to toxic gases during the course of their duties. Smoke inhalation can produce adverse effects in the upper airways and lungs from the heat alone. Carbon monoxide results from incomplete combustion of flammable materials. Hydrogen cyanide and irritant gases, such as phosgene, are pyrolysis products of certain plastics. The history and clinical course of this patient suggests that he was exposed to a slowly acting pulmonary irritant, such as the oxides of nitrogen (e.g., NO or NO_2, but not the anesthetic N_2O). These gases are slowly hydrolyzed by moisture in the respiratory tract to form the proximal irritant, nitric acid (HNO_3). The full-blown reaction in this case developed over the 24 hours after exposure.

Actually, the identity of the causative agent is not critical, since acute noncardiogenic pulmonary edema is treated much the same irrespective of the agent involved. Immediate measures would include oxygen therapy, bed rest, and mechanical ventilation if necessary. If bronchospasm develops, then administration of theophylline or inhaled beta-2 agonists may also be helpful. Although there is little evidence that it does any good after exposure has occurred, corticosteroids have been given in an effort to reduce the inflammatory response. Antibiotics would be indicated in the event of secondary bacterial infection.

CHAPTER 61

ALCOHOLS

Related Readings

Clark et al: Chapter 26, pp. 292-298
Craig and Stitzel: Chapter 36
Gilman et al: Chapter 18
Katzung: Chapter 21

Key Concepts

- Management of methanol intoxication
- Management of ethanol intoxication
- Management of ethanol withdrawal

QUESTIONS

1. An automobile mechanic was working on an engine in his repair shop on a hot August day. He was thirsty, but had run out of iced tea. He noticed a large open bottle of Sprite™ on the next workbench, and decided that his friend wouldn't mind if he had a bit. He drank thirstily from the bottle, and only after he had swallowed several large mouthfuls did he notice that the clear liquid was not Sprite™ at all, but rather a funny-tasting liquid that made his mouth burn. It smelled like a solvent they used in the shop to degrease engine parts.

He went back to work, but his friends noticed him a few minutes later because he appeared to act drunk. This was unusual, since his friends knew that he never drank ethanol. When they took him to the emergency room about 2 hours after the ingestion, he also complained of dim vision. What do you think he drank? How would you confirm the diagnosis? How would you treat the ingestion?

2. A 19-year-old young man was attending a fraternity party to celebrate the initiation of new pledges into the fraternity. Each pledge was urged to drink a quart of vodka. What effects would you predict would result from the rapid ingestion of this amount of ethanol?

3. A 57-year-old business executive had grown accustomed to drinking almost one quart of bourbon each day. He started off his day with one or two drinks before breakfast, and then continued drinking throughout the day. One morning while shaving, he noted the onset of crushing chest pain radiating to his jaw and arm. He was taken to the hospital, and admitted to the coronary care unit with a diagnosis of acute myocardial infarction. Within 24 hours he became tremulous and anxious. In the hours that followed, he became more anxious, and began to have visual hallucinations. During his third hospital day, he experienced one grand-mal seizure and was noted to be febrile, with a resting tachycardia, increased blood pressure, and sweating.

What do you think was happening to the patient? Is this condition dangerous? How should it be treated?

ANSWERS

1. A degreasing solvent that can produce signs and symptoms of ethanol intoxication followed by dimness of vision is methanol or wood alcohol. Other data that would support this diagnosis include rapid breathing and hyperventilation; blood gases and electrolytes showing a respiratory alkalosis and a metabolic acidosis with a low bicarbonate and increased anion gap; a gap between the measured and calculated serum osmolality; and a high serum methanol level (a specific test that may take several hours to return).

Most of these problems can be traced to the fact that methanol itself is an alcohol that produces intoxication similar to that caused by ethanol. However, methanol is metabolized by alcohol dehydrogenase to formaldehyde, which is then further metabolized by aldehyde dehydrogenase to formic acid. It is likely that the latter is responsible for the damage to the optic nerve, as well as contributing to the metabolic acidosis.

There are several steps to be considered in the management of this patient. In addition to the general supportive care given to all intoxicated or poisoned patients, he should be given ethanol by either the oral or intravenous route. The ethanol serves as a competitive inhibitor of the enzyme alcohol dehydrogenase, thereby slowing the metabolism of methanol to formaldehyde. Methanol, formaldehyde, and formic acid are all small, water-soluble molecules that are rapidly cleared by hemodialysis. In serious intoxications, prompt institution of hemodialysis can be beneficial and even lifesaving. Finally, usual supportive care should not be overlooked. For example, if the patient manifests a serious metabolic acidosis, he should be given sodium bicarbonate intravenously until a normal blood pH is restored. The dose may have to be repeated at frequent intervals.

Intoxication with this chemical illustrates that the physician must be concerned with the toxin's metabolites as well as with the parent toxin itself.

2. If ingested over a relatively short period of time (e.g., a few hours or less), this is a potentially lethal dose of ethanol for an adult human. A person unaccustomed to drinking may be able to eliminate (metabolize) only 7 to 10 g of ethanol each hour. Thus rapid ingestion overwhelms the patient's ability to metabolize the compound, and the serum alcohol level rapidly rises beyond the lower limits of legal intoxication (100 mg/dl or 1000 mg/L) towards more life-threatening serum concentrations. If the stomach was otherwise empty at the time of ingestion, absorption may be extremely rapid, and death may occur quickly from respiratory or circulatory failure.

Otherwise, the patient will still progress rapidly through the familiar stages of emotional lability, impaired motor coordination, sensory disturbances, peripheral vascular collapse and respiratory depression. If the patient vomits while he is obtunded, there is the further danger of aspiration pneumonitis and death from an associated pneumonitis. If the patient passes out in a cool (e.g., inside room) or cold (e.g., park bench) environment, hypothermia is an additional risk. Severe ethanol intoxication is a true medical emergency that again may require extra-corporeal hemodialysis.

When you review this case, you may think that it is unnecessary to be familiar with the presentation and management of severe ethanol intoxication. However, each year there continues to be a disturbing number of deaths on college campuses (and even at high school parties) because of severe ethanol intoxications. It is essential to realize that severe ethanol intoxication includes adverse effects much more serious than simply "blacking out."

3. This patient is exhibiting the classic syndrome of alcohol withdrawal in a physically dependent person. The withdrawal syndrome includes a spectrum of symptoms and signs ranging from mild and early presentations (anxiety, tremor, craving alcohol) to more severe signs (agitation, hallucinations) to a full-blown toxic delirium with sympathetic autonomic excess (delirium tremens). Withdrawal seizures ("rum fits") may occur as well.

Unlike the abstinence syndrome resulting from opioid withdrawal, which is unpleasant but not necessarily life-threatening, withdrawal from alcohol (or barbiturates) initiates a potentially dangerous reaction because of the possibility of violent convulsive episodes. While alcohol withdrawal is unpleasant, it may become life-threatening if it occurs in a patient with a concomitant severe illness such as gastrointestinal bleeding, pancreatitis, pneumonia, or heart disease. This patient would be at considerable risk of developing angina (or even extending his myocardial infarction) if he developed full-blown delirium tremens.

The treatment (or better still, the prophylaxis) of the alcohol withdrawal state involves the substituting of a moderately long-acting drug that can replace the ethanol. Such a drug is said to exhibit cross-dependence and cross-tolerance with ethanol. Although barbiturates have been used in the past for this purpose, the drugs of choice today would be medium- to long-acting benzodiazepines, such as diazepam, chlordiazepoxide, or lorazepam. Although each of these drugs has certain advantages and disadvantages, lorazepam is considered by many to be the drug of choice because it can be easily given by three routes (orally, intravenously, or intramuscularly), has a shorter half-life of elimination (about 12 hours), and has more predictable elimination in patients with alcoholic liver disease. Once a patient is stabilized with one of these drugs, the dosage can then be gradually reduced over several days to gently wean the patient off the benzodiazepine and moderate the intense withdrawal reaction.

CHAPTER 62

DRUG AND SUBSTANCE ABUSE

Related Readings

Clark et al: Chapter 30
Craig and Stitzel: Chapter 44
Gilman et al: Chapter 23
Katzung: Chapter 30

Key Concepts

- Cocaine abuse
- Nicotine abuse
- Opioid abuse

QUESTIONS

1. A 21-year-old college student and his friends are celebrating his recent draft by the NFL. His friends encourage him to smoke several pieces of crack. Several minutes after he begins smoking, he starts to feel a rush of euphoria and power. Several minutes after that, his friends note that he suddenly slumps to the ground and appears to have a grand mal seizure. His friends bring him to a nearby emergency room, where he appears to be pulseless and apneic. The initial cardiac rhythm taken shows him to be in ventricular fibrillation. Unfortunately, he is unable to be resuscitated. What happened?

2. A 43-year-old secretary develops chronic bronchitis and decides that she must give up her habit of smoking two packs of cigarettes each day. She decides to switch to a low-tar cigarette, but finds that she is smoking more cigarettes each day. The same thing happens when she switches to a thinner, "feminine" cigarette. When she decides to simply stop smoking "cold turkey," she becomes extremely agitated and nervous, and develops severe headaches. Why does she find it so hard to stop smoking?

3. A 29-year-old nurse finds that she has ready access to parenteral formulations of various opioids, such as morphine and meperidine, which she is supposed to inject into patients. She finds that she can inject one-half the prescribed dose into the patient, and "pocket" the difference. Since most of the prescribed injections are into intravenous tubing, she can take the prepackaged syringes home and they are still sterile. She finds that she has been taking more and more injections recently in an attempt to achieve the same relaxing effect.

She appears to be functioning well at work, although at times her behavior seems sluggish or inappropriate. Her absenteeism is up a bit, but none of her colleagues suspect her problem. Her coffee breaks become more frequent and longer. One day she is forced to stay home from work because of a severely sprained ankle, and she uses up her supply of opioids. What do you think might happen?

ANSWERS

1. The initial intoxicating effects of cocaine, especially when "crack" is rapidly absorbed via inhalational or intravenous routes, include a rush of euphoria and a feeling of power that is strongly reinforcing, and which can lead to the compulsive abuse of cocaine. Cocaine is particularly dangerous in the form of crack, because the free base is so rapidly absorbed through the lungs. Very severe systemic sympathomimetic signs and symptoms follow quickly, because cocaine blocks the re-uptake of norepinephrine at adrenergic nerve terminals. Both alpha-adrenergic and beta-adrenergic receptor-mediated effects of norepinephrine are strongly potentiated since the effect of cocaine is on the presynaptic nerve terminal. The postsynaptic receptors are unaffected, but they are flooded with unusually large concentrations of the transmitter. Hence, blood pressure may rise abruptly and to dangerous levels because of the activation of alpha-receptors. At the same time the beta-receptors on the heart are activated, resulting in tachycardia.

Other severe signs of intoxication can also include headache, intractable grand mal seizures, hypoxemia, refractory or lethal ventricular arrhythmias, myocardial infarction, and myocarditis with repeated use.

Tolerance probably develops to cocaine, especially after the use of the free base (crack). Dependence, both psychologic and physiologic, also can develop quickly. After dependence occurs, sudden discontinuation of cocaine use results in a withdrawal state similar to that seen during withdrawal from amphetamines. Addiction, in a social or behavioral sense, definitely occurs, with addicts devoting larger portions of their time, money, and lives to obtaining and using the drug. Finally, the medical consequences of this addiction can be severe, ranging from perforation of the nasal septum to sudden death.

2. After many years of debate, most authorities (including the surgeon general) now regard nicotine as a truly addictive substance. This woman has become dependent on a given level of nicotine intake. The acute intoxication associated with smoking nicotine is minimal, and tolerance to nicotine has not been proven. However, psychologic and physiologic dependence is clearly a factor in this case.

Both the low-tar cigarettes and the longer, thinner "feminine" cigarettes provide either decreased amounts or increased filtering of both tar and nicotine. Neither cigarette provided the dose of nicotine to which she had become accustomed. Therefore she developed a mild withdrawal reaction, and sought to increase her nicotine intake by smoking more cigarettes. When she abruptly stopped smoking, she developed a more severe withdrawal reaction. Her agitation and nervousness were probably the result of central nervous system deprivation of nicotine. The headache may have been caused by nicotine deprivation at sympathetic ganglia where the stimulation at low doses leads to vasoconstriction. In the absence of nicotine there may be dilatation of meningeal arteries, resulting in headache.

3. When her supply of opioids has been exhausted and the acute effects of the last dose (euphoria or rush, followed by sedation or even coma) wear off, she will begin to experience an opioid withdrawal syndrome within a few hours. It is clear that opioids cause the development of tolerance, psychologic and physiologic dependence, and a withdrawal syndrome.

Many of the signs and symptoms of the withdrawal syndrome resemble overactivity of the sympathetic nervous system or hyperthyroidism. She will experience lacrimation, a watery discharge from the nose, yawning, and sweating. Her sleep will be restless. She will experience weakness, piloerection (gooseflesh), nausea and vomiting, muscle aches and involuntary movements, hyperpnea, fever, and hypertension. This acute withdrawal reaction may last for a week or more. It is not particularly dangerous, but she will have an overwhelming desire to obtain more opioids to stop it. A secondary phase with somewhat different signs and symptoms may last for as long as 6 months. If she obtains more opioids or is admitted to a methadone substitution (maintenance) program, her withdrawal syndrome would be terminated, although she would not have been "detoxified."

Opioids obviously can lead to addiction, with the addict spending a great deal of time, effort, and money to obtain his or her "fix." Addicts can range from intravenous abusers nodding off in alleys to respected professionals who may be very difficult to detect, especially if they have easy access to the drugs themselves. Sometimes only gradual changes in their behavior tips off coworkers to the problem. Problems associated with addiction include social problems (crime, prison), economic problems (loss of work), and medical problems (overdose, endocarditis, hepatitis and AIDS from sharing needles, pulmonary edema, constipation, and death).

CHAPTER 63

MANAGEMENT OF THE POISONED PATIENT

Related Readings

Clark et al: Chapter 62; Chapter 29, p. 325; Chapter 31, pp. 368-370
Craig and Stitzel: Chapter 8; Chapter 42, pp. 589-591; Chapter 43, pp.599-600
Gilman et al: Chapter 68; Chapter 22, pp. 509-510; Chapter 29, p. 694
Katzung: Chapter 62; Chapter 29, p. 346; Chapter 34, pp. 408-409

Key Concepts

- General principles of management of the intoxicated patient
- Applications of those principles to a specific case: intoxication with Percocet™ (acetaminophen/oxycodone combination)

QUESTIONS

1. Patients may come to the emergency room with an accidental or deliberate overdose with either prescription or over-the-counter drugs. In addition, other patients may have been accidently poisoned or intoxicated with a non-drug product, such as a petroleum distillate, insecticide, or bleach. As different as these patients are from one another, a certain common and rational approach can be followed with all of these patients. What are the essential elements of such an approach?

2. A 24-year-old waitress was very depressed, and she decided to end her life by ingesting 50 Percocet™ tablets. Her sister found her in a coma, and took her to the emergency room. The diagnosis was suggested by the presence of coma, shallow respirations, constricted pupils, and the empty bottle found near the bedside. She was given several ampules of Narcan™ and rapidly awakened. After 15 minutes, she was sent home.

Her sister brought her back within 1 hour because she had lapsed back into a coma. Once again she received Narcan™ with good results, and she was sent back home. This time she became sleepy, but did not become comatose. However, 2 days later she again returned to the emergency department complaining of yellow eyes, dark urine, and soreness in her right upper quadrant.

How would you evaluate the overall treatment of this patient's intoxication?

ANSWERS

1. Although you must begin to develop the knowledge base to treat common intoxications, it is probably more important to develop an overall plan for treating any type of intoxication. There is no way that anyone can memorize the characteristics and management of all types of intoxications, so a useful general approach to these situations is essential.

When the patient is initially examined, the first job is to stabilize the patient's condition. This involves maintaining a patent airway, ensuring that ventilation is adequate, and supporting circulation if necessary. In addition, hypotension and seizures are frequent problems that must be treated. Since coma can be caused by drug-induced hypoglycemia, it is probably a good idea to send a blood sample for glucose determination, and give 25 g of dextrose intravenously. Other supportive measures that are often given to any comatose patient include administration of thiamine and Narcan™, an opioid antagonist with the generic name naloxone.

Next, you must quickly evaluate the patient by performing an abbreviated history and physical examination, and sending a few pertinent laboratory tests. From these clues, you must try to deductively reason what drugs or poisons, if any, are responsible for the patient's condition.

Then you must try to remove any unabsorbed poison. For topical exposure, washing the skin is necessary. Since most drugs are taken by mouth, you must either induce vomiting, or pump out (lavage) the stomach. It is dangerous to induce vomiting in a comatose patient, and you may have to intubate the patient's trachea to protect the airway before inserting a nasogastric tube into the stomach.

Next, some drugs or poisons require specific treatments, and a few require the administration of specific antidotes. For example, intoxication with carbon monoxide requires the administration of oxygen, whereas iron intoxication may require the administration of deferoxamine, a chelating agent.

It is occasionally useful to try to hasten the elimination of the drug or poison involved. This should be attempted only if the potential benefits outweigh the potential risks of the procedure. This can sometimes be accomplished by adjusting the urinary pH or flow rate, or by instituting hemodialysis or hemoperfusion, or even by giving activated charcoal by mouth to diminish enterohepatic recirculation.

Finally, you must be aware that some poisons cause late complications. For example, iron intoxication causes severe enterocolitis and shock hours or days after the initial ingestion.

You will see in the next problem how some of these principles were applied in an actual case.

2. Although this young woman was comatose when brought to the hospital, her ventilation and circulation were adequate, and there were no life-threatening problems such as seizures or arrhythmias that required specific steps for stabilization. She should have had a blood sample sent for glucose determination and received intravenous dextrose and thiamine.

A quick assessment of the patient included her history (the empty bottle of Percocet™) and physical examination (coma, shallow respirations, pinpoint pupils), which suggested the diagnosis of opioid overdose. In fact, Percocet™ tablets contain both acetaminophen (325 mg) and oxycodone (5 mg), an opioid.

This likely diagnosis, along with the fact that most comatose patients should receive naloxone, led the physician to administer increasing doses of intravenous naloxone. This opioid antagonist blocked the central nervous system depressant effects of oxycodone, and caused the patient to wake up.

However, the patient's stomach contents were never evacuated, and the patient continued to absorb the acetaminophen and oxycodone remaining in her gastrointestinal tract. For this reason, as well as the fact that the half-life of naloxone is shorter than the half-life of oxycodone, she lapsed back into a coma shortly after she was released from the hospital. A second dose of naloxone revived her, and she was again discharged, still without having had her stomach evacuated.

It is true that there is no practical way of enhancing the clearance of either acetaminophen or oxycodone. However, the treating physician simply forgot that Percocet™ contains acetaminophen as well as oxycodone, and in fact this ingestion of 50 tablets is a very large and dangerous ingestion of acetaminophen. Had the physician recognized this, he should have evacuated the stomach and sent a blood sample to measure the amount of acetaminophen in the circulation. If it were sufficiently high, then he should have instituted therapy with oral N-acetylcysteine, an antidote useful in preventing the potentially severe late hepatotoxicity caused by acetaminophen (more specifically, by toxic metabolites of acetaminophen). Unfortunately, when the young woman returned the next day, she was suffering from massive hepatic necrosis caused by the unrecognized and untreated acetaminophen toxicity.

This case illustrates how important it is to keep a general approach to such cases in mind, even if the case and its treatment seem very simple at the beginning.

SECTION TEN

MISCELLANEOUS TOPICS

CHAPTER 64

DRUGS ACTING ON THE GASTROINTESTINAL TRACT AND UTERUS

Related Readings

Clark et al: Chapter 24, p. 255; Chapter 41, pp. 519-522; Chapter 21, pp. 218-219
Craig and Stitzel: Chapter 69, pp. 982-987; Chapter 13, pp. 182-183
Gilman et al: Chapter 5, p. 108; Chapter 42, pp. 980-987; Chapter 39, pp. 931-940
Katzung: Chapter 66; Chapter 15, pp. 195-199

Key Concepts

- Metoclopramide: actions and adverse effects
- Antacids: actions and adverse effects
- Ergot alkaloids: effects on the uterus

QUESTIONS

1. A 50-year-old man with diabetes mellitus was bothered by reflux esophagitis—symptoms of acid refluxing upwards into the esophagus and causing substernal burning. Further evaluation of this problem indicated that he had diabetic gastroparesis—a failure of the stomach to empty normally. His physician recommended that he take a drug called metoclopramide to ameliorate both problems. How could one drug help both conditions?

He began taking the drug, and on the second day he suddenly developed a painful spasm of the muscles in his neck and trunk, with his head painfully twisted towards the right. Also, he seemed to be staring upwards, and couldn't bring his eyes down to maintain a level gaze. What happened?

2. A 63-year-old man had occasional "indigestion" after eating large meals, and treated himself with one tablespoon of baking soda. This usually produced a large belch within a few minutes, and usually relieved his sense of indigestion. Over several months, he noticed that he was developing a different type of abdominal discomfort. About 1 hour after eating a meal, he noted a gnawing pain in his epigastrium that tended to persist. This same pain often awakened him around 3 AM. He began treating himself with the same remedy, baking soda. Although this usually made him feel better, he found that he was taking one or two tablespoons up to eight times every day to relieve the pain. Over several weeks, he noticed that his ankles began to swell. What do you think of his therapeutic trial?

3. During childbirth, if there is significant hemorrhage from the uterus after the placenta has been delivered, an injection of ergonovine maleate causes uterine contraction and helps reduce uterine bleeding. However, if this drug or another ergot alkaloid is given during labor in an effort to stimulate uterine contractions, the results are often adverse and can include fetal or maternal death. Why does the same drug, causing the "same effect," work so well in one situation and so poorly in another?

ANSWERS

1. Metoclopramide has cholinomimetic activity at muscarinic receptors, particularly in the gastrointestinal tract, but it is not a direct-acting agonist. It seems to sensitize intestinal smooth muscle to the actions of acetylcholine. Its stimulant effects on the gastrointestinal tract hasten esophageal clearance, enhance the competency of the lower esophageal sphincter, and accelerate gastric emptying. These actions provide effective relief for heartburn of esophageal reflux, particularly in patients with marginal gastric motor activity as in diabetic gastroparesis. Metoclopramide also shortens the bowel transit time.

At the same time, the drug is a potent dopamine receptor blocker, particularly in the central nervous system. This additional property is probably responsible for its antiemetic activity. In addition, this antagonistic activity is responsible for one of its side effects, which is shared by many antipsychotic drugs, namely acute dystonic reactions (such as the typical one experienced by this patient). The timing of the reaction so quickly after starting therapy and the specific nature of the reaction suggest that this extrapyramidal reaction is not the more serious and potentially irreversible tardive dyskinesia. An acute dystonic reaction can be rapidly terminated by the administration of either diphenhydramine or benztropine. The patient may respond to a lowering of the dosage and not have a recurrence with continued therapy.

2. The clinical presentation of this patient's new epigastric gnawing pain strongly suggests the diagnosis of peptic ulcer disease, as does the timing of the pain after meals and in the early morning. Satisfactory pain relief and healing can be achieved with various classes of drugs, including oral H_2-receptor antagonists and oral nonsystemic antacid preparations (e.g., aluminum or magnesium hydroxides).

Unfortunately, this patient selected an antacid that is well absorbed and has systemic effects—sodium bicarbonate ($NaHCO_3$). Although it provided relief for his mild indigestion early on (by neutralizing hydrochloric acid and forming carbon dioxide), it became increasingly ineffective as the ulcer disease progressed, in part because its buffering effects are so transient. Because of the larger doses he was taking as the ulcer worsened, he continued to absorb large amounts of sodium (leading to fluid retention and ankle edema) and bicarbonate (leading to a systemic alkalosis).

He must stop taking sodium bicarbonate and switch to more appropriate ulcer treatment as mentioned above. The salt and water retention should improve after the sodium bicarbonate ingestion ceases, although this could be hastened by the administration of a diuretic.

3. All of the naturally occurring ergot alkaloids are oxytocic, which means that they increase the motor activity of the uterus in terms of both force and frequency of contractions. This effect increases in intensity as the dosage is increased, and it can ultimately result in a sustained contracture. Thus, they are not suited for the induction or intensification of labor. In fact, ergot poisoning in pregnant women during the epidemics of the Middle Ages often resulted in abortion.*

This oxytocic action can be exploited therapeutically, however, in the postpartum phase to help expel the placenta and control endometrial bleeding. The effect on bleeding may partly result from a direct vasoconstrictor action as well as the increased uterine tone. Of all the ergot alkaloids, ergonovine seems to be the most selective in its effects on the uterus. Thus, if an ergot preparation is required in this situation, ergonovine is usually the one that is prescribed.

*Poisoning resulted from the consumption of bread made with grain contaminated with ergot-producing fungi.

CHAPTER 65

EMETICS AND ANTIEMETICS

Related Readings

Clark et al: Chapter 62, pp. 731-732; Chapter 12, p. 117; Chapter 20, p. 208-209; Chapter 24, pp. 252-256
Craig and Stitzel: Chapter 69, pp. 981-983
Gilman et al: Chapter 68, pp. 1599-1600; Chapter 19, pp. 411-412; Chapter 7, p. 143; Chapter 26, p. 624
Katzung: Chapter 62, p. 744; Chapter 7, p. 78; Chapter 15, p. 189; Chapter 27, p. 319

Key Concepts

- Drugs used to produce emesis, and their adverse effects
- Different classes of drugs with antiemetic effects

QUESTIONS

1. Drugs that cause emesis are rarely given. However, there is one fairly common situation in which such a drug would be useful, for instance, in the case of an 18-month-old toddler who gets into his mother's bottle of iron supplements and swallows quite a few. The mother calls from home to say that the child is awake and alert; you calculate that the amount of iron ingested could result in a serious case of iron intoxication. What would you suggest the mother do? Should she keep any medicine at home for this purpose? Are there any potential side effects of this medicine if taken in excess?

2. Many different drugs from several different classes have proved to be useful in reducing episodes of nausea and vomiting. Which drugs might you try first for the following patients with vomiting problems? What are their proposed mechanisms of action?

1. A 17-year-old boy about to receive his third round of chemotherapy to treat his lymphoma
2. A 25-year-old woman who develops mild motion sickness on an airplane
3. A 43-year-old man who must cross the English channel, but who knows that he develops violent nausea and vomiting while on the water
4. A 23-year-old student who develops severe nausea and vomiting during the course of a viral gastroenteritis.

ANSWERS

1. In this type of case, an emetic drug could prevent serious poisoning by preventing further disintegration of the tablets in the stomach and the absorption of toxic amounts of iron. Syrup of ipecac is a reasonably safe and effective drug that causes vomiting by causing a local irritant effect directly on the gastrointestinal tract, and also by stimulating the chemoreceptor trigger zone in the brainstem. This central effect is caused by two alkaloids, emetine and cephaeline. The syrup may be purchased without a prescription, and should be kept in any home with toddlers or children for just this purpose. In many communities, the local pharmacists distribute the drug free of charge as a promotional device during National Poison Prevention Week.

Parents should always be advised to call their physician or poison control center before using the drug, because there are situations where induced vomiting can make things worse (e.g., ingestion of a caustic substance). If syrup of ipecac is taken in excess, the vomiting may be dangerously prolonged, leading to fluid and electrolyte imbalances. Also, the alkaloid emetine is cardiotoxic in high concentrations. Be sure not to confuse syrup of ipecac with fluid extract of ipecac, which is 14 times more concentrated, and which has caused some deaths.

2. A number of different classes of drugs have demonstrated antiemetic effects. In many cases, exact mechanisms of action have not been firmly established, but empirical evidence has suggested that certain types of drugs are likely to be more effective in certain clinical situations.

The vomiting secondary to cancer chemotherapy is particularly distressing. Drugs that have proven to be effective in this situation include antipsychotic agents, such as prochlorperazine or droperidol; corticosteroids, such as dexamethasone; sedatives, such as lorazepam; and metoclopramide. Recently, there has been great interest in the use of the marijuana cannabinoids, such as Δ^9-tetrahydrocannabinol, to control these episodes. These preparations are still not generally available, but FDA approval may come in the near future. Its mechanism of action is unknown.

For the adult with a history of mild motion sickness, you might recommend that she premedicate herself before take off with dimenhydrinate, an antihistamine that depresses the sensitivity of the vestibular apparatus. The more extreme form of motion sickness caused by ocean travel might best be managed with transdermal patches of scopolamine. Although both drugs have anticholinergic properties, their exact mechanisms of antiemetic activity are unknown.

The severe nausea and vomiting secondary to viral gastroenteritis might respond to the antiemetic, antipsychotic drugs, such as prochlorperazine or promethazine, which block dopamine receptors.

As you might expect, each class of antiemetic agents has its own profile of side effects. Thus, the rational use of antiemetics to maximize benefit and minimize toxicity is often a clinical challenge.

CHAPTER 66

DRUG DEVELOPMENT AND DRUG ADVERTISING

Related Readings

Clark et al: Chapter 5
Craig and Stitzel: Chapter 9
Gilman et al: Chapter 3
Katzung: Chapter 4

Key Concepts

- Difficulties and costs of new drug development
- Understanding drug advertisements
- The relationship between medical students and drug companies

QUESTIONS

1. In your basic pharmacology laboratory, you make the interesting discovery that a chemical used to inhibit the P450 enzyme system seems to cause a profound increase in the force of contraction of the heart. This chemical has been around for more than 30 years, is widely available from chemical supply companies, and has never been marketed for any medicinal purpose. You try to interest one of the pharmaceutical houses in further testing of this agent that you have "discovered." From the point of view of the drug company, what are the issues involved? What is the company looking at in terms of experiments needed, cost, time, and likelihood of "payback"?

2. A new nonsteroidal anti-inflammatory drug is approved by the FDA for the treatment of rheumatoid arthritis. As the advertisements for the new drug begin to be seen in leading medical journals, one ad catches your eye. It says that the new drug, ArthroFix™, is "unsurpassed in the management of arthritis pain." This message, and the smiling patient who is now obviously free of pain, make you eager to prescribe this new drug for your next patient with painful rheumatoid arthritis. What do you think this ad is "really" saying, based on your knowledge of similar advertisements?

3. Drug manufacturing companies may offer a number of inducements to medical students and physicians to encourage prescribers to think well of the company name or to use a specific drug. Consider the following practices: printing free books and teaching materials for medical students; providing free stethoscopes engraved with the company name; providing free black bags embossed with the company name; providing free pens, clips, and cards stamped with drug names; providing free pizzas during house-staff lunches, with the understanding that the sales representative has 10 minutes to introduce a new product; sponsoring guest lecturers to visit a medical school and to deliver medical grand rounds; sponsoring free seminars at exclusive Florida resorts, with all expenses paid, to discuss the pharmacologic management of a specific disease. Will such activities encourage rational prescribing? Who pays for such activities?

ANSWERS

1. The preliminary testing required before the FDA could approve the drug as being "safe and effective" could cost as much as 80 to 100 million dollars, and take as long as 5 to 10 years after the drug is initially "discovered." There are an enormous number of animal studies of efficacy and toxicity (preclinical studies) that must be completed before a drug company can even apply for an Investigational New Drug exemption (IND) to test the drug in humans. Then, several years of clinical testing follow before the company can apply to the FDA for consideration of a New Drug Application (NDA). At any step along this path, the drug may be abandoned because of lack of efficacy, excessive toxicity, or both. No drug company would be willing to make such a staggering investment of time, effort, and resources unless its interests and its ability to recover some of these costs through profits could be protected by an exclusive patent.

Since most drug patents cover newly-discovered chemicals, a company is not apt to be interested in your drug, no matter how good it might be as a positive inotropic agent. As many as 5,000 to 10,000 new compounds may be synthesized, tested, and discarded for each successful drug, so the odds are heavily stacked against any single compound making the grade. Even a drug that is highly effective as an inotropic agent may be rejected on the grounds of its toxicity. However, the financial rewards for successfully developing a new drug can be enormous, and this fact keeps the drug industry profitable, productive, and interested in discovering and testing new products.

2. The advertisement is not so remarkable for what it says as for what it does *not* say. The smiling patient and the fact that this drug is "unsurpassed" at relieving pain are in its favor. However, the ad does not say how this new drug compares in terms of effectiveness, safety, and cost to other drugs that are already available to treat the pain of rheumatoid arthritis. Other useful comparative information of secondary importance might include: how often the drug has to be given to produce maximum benefit, whether or not it can be given by mouth, whether it has any unusual or severe adverse effects, and many other features that might influence a rational decision about whether to use it in preference to some other drug.

Since none of this information appears in the ad, you might interpret the statement "unsurpassed in the management of arthritis pain" as meaning that the new drug is essentially comparable to older nonsteroidal anti-inflammatory drugs already available—including aspirin. Remember, unsurpassed does not mean "superior to," it means "as good as but not better than." Since it is a new drug that may have dangerous side effects that have not yet been recognized because it has not been given to a large group of patients, you have at least one good reason to avoid it and no compelling reason to use it just yet.

3. Many of these inducements are not likely to lead to rational prescribing. Some of these programs (e.g., publishing excellent educational material for medical students, helping to sponsor quality educational programs) represent useful services, although others would argue that such material still represents advertising for the company name, if not for a specific product.

Although many physicians and students say that they would not be personally swayed by such things as free pens, calipers, trips, or lunches, sales figures tend to suggest that these practices are highly successful. It is probably true that there is no such thing as a free lunch. The costs for these programs are ultimately passed on to the patient in terms of increased costs for the drug itself.

Individual physicians, as well as scientific and professional societies, are increasingly looking for ways to optimize interactions with pharmaceutical companies. There is little doubt that in matters of basic research, clinical research, and educational activities, physicians and drug companies can often work together constructively. It is also clear that when physicians prescribe drugs irrationally, patient care will often suffer. In the final analysis, each doctor and medical student must determine how to best structure his or her relationship with drug companies so that the benefits of these associations are not diminished by temptations to practice irrational therapy.

CHAPTER 67

PRESCRIPTION WRITING

Related Readings

Clark et al: Chapter 64
Craig and Stitzel: Chapter 7, pp. 96-110; Chapter 9, pp. 127-133
Gilman et al: Appendix I, pp. 1651-1662
Katzung: Chapter 69, pp. 802-806

Key Concepts

- Essential parts of the written drug prescription
- Special considerations when prescribing controlled substances

QUESTIONS

1. There are several essential parts to any written prescription. Discuss the following prescription written by one of the authors:

Patient: David Nierenberg
Rx: Amoxil
Disp: 4 oz.
Sig: Take as directed
Signed: David Nierenberg, M.D.

2. You accept an internship at a hospital located in a small town. One night you return home from work and find that your dog has many porcupine quills stuck in his nose. You decide to remove them yourself, and call the town pharmacy to order a prescription of parenteral morphine sulfate solution for your dog, with two refills if necessary. Since this is a controlled substance, you give your hospital DEA number over the phone. Should the pharmacist honor this prescription?

ANSWERS

1. There are eight essential parts to a written prescription that clarify it and make it more likely to be dispensed and taken properly. These eight parts are over and above the requirement that the drug and dosage you prescribe are correct, and that you have written legibly. Unfortunately, the sample prescription shown on the previous page has many deficiencies.

First, you should give enough details about the patient so that the pharmacist knows who is receiving the prescription. Include the patient's age and address as well. This will alert the pharmacist to the fact that you are prescribing for a child who happens to have the same name as the prescribing physician. Also, be sure to write the date of the prescription. The pharmacist is unlikely to fill a prescription that is very old; and the patient will know when he looks at the bottle how old the prescription really is (old prescriptions should be thrown out to avoid confusion).

It is traditional to include the symbol Rx, which is the abbreviation for recipe (Latin, *take thou*). This serves to introduce the next part of the prescription, a clear statement as to which drug and which specific formulation you wish to prescribe. In this case, you would order a pediatric oral suspension, since the patient is only 6 years old. Be sure to specify the exact strength of the solution, or the exact size of the tablet or capsule. Generally, you should order drugs by their generic names, since such preparations are usually as good (similar bioavailability and peak plasma concentrations) as the more expensive trade name versions, and usually cost your patient less.

You must then tell the pharmacist how to dispense the drug. For an oral (liquid) suspension, you should calculate the volume of the suspension needed, and order it in milliliters (ml). This is the only currently accepted unit of volume (not cc's or ounces). Units of mass would be milligrams or grams, not ounces or grains. You must then give the pharmacist directions for labeling the prescription. The label should include detailed directions, including how to administer the drug, how often, for how long, and for what indication.

Finally, you must not only sign the prescription, but also print your name and include your telephone number and address. This helps the pharmacist or patient reach you with any questions that may come up. You must also mention whether the prescription can be refilled, and if so, how many times. In this case, you do *not* want the prescription to be refilled.

A better prescription would look like this:
Patient: David Nierenberg Jr, age 6, Lebanon, NH
Date: July 1, 1988
Rx: Amoxicillin pediatric oral suspension, 125 mg/5 ml
Dispense: 250 ml with measuring teaspoon (5 ml)
Label: Take 7.5 ml (1½ teaspoons) by mouth three times daily for 10 days, for inner ear infection. Shake well each time before using.
Refills: Do not refill
Signed: David Nierenberg, M.D. (with printed name and office phone)

By writing legibly, avoiding old-fashioned units and Latin abbreviations, and writing a complete prescription, you will minimize the chances of the patient or pharmacist making a serious or even fatal error.

2. It is certainly understandable that you wish to relieve your dog's pain while you remove those porcupine quills. It is likely that a veterinarian would have the facilities to do this more quickly and painlessly. However, should you try to obtain this prescription, you would immediately discover some major problems.

First, morphine is an opioid (narcotic) with strong abuse potential. Therefore, it is a controlled substance and has strict laws governing its prescription and dispensing. Since it is a Schedule II drug (with legitimate therapeutic uses but the greatest liability for abuse), it may not be prescribed over the phone (except in rare situations that will not be discussed here). Also, no refills are permitted. In addition, in many states, a physician may not prescribe any controlled substance for either himself or a member of his immediate family.

As an unlicensed intern, your DEA (Drug Enforcement Administration) number provided by the hospital can only be used in the hospital in conjunction with usual hospital duties. It can not be used by an intern in any other way. Finally, just as veterinarians are not allowed to prescribe drugs for people, physicians are not allowed to prescribe drugs for animals. All in all, you would do better to take your dog to the veterinarian right away.

CHAPTER 68

INTRODUCTION TO CLINICAL PHARMACOLOGY

Related Readings

Clark et al: Chapter 5; Chapter 16, pp. 165-170; Chapter 52
Craig and Stitzel: Chapter 13, pp. 183-192; Chapter 46, pp. 641-648
Gilman et al: Chapter 3, pp. 49-65; Chapter 9, pp. 192-201; Chapter 49, pp. 1095-1114
Katzung: Chapter 9, pp. 99-104; Chapter 47

Key Concepts

- Key steps in the process of rational prescribing
- Two important principles of rational drug therapy

QUESTIONS

1. A 45-year-old woman came to an emergency room, complaining of several mildly pruritic hives that developed on her chest and arms a few minutes after she was stung by a bee. She had no complaints of wheezing, shortness of breath, or swelling of her tongue or lips. The only remarkable factor in her history was that she took propranolol 20 mg four times daily to treat "palpitations." The physician in the emergency room administered epinephrine 0.3 mg subcutaneously to treat her allergic reaction. Within a few minutes her blood pressure climbed from 120/80 mm Hg up to 225/125 mm Hg, while her pulse slowed slightly. She complained of a severe headache, and then noted that her speech became slurred and she felt weak on the right side of her body.

Over the next few minutes, her blood pressure returned to normal. However, she was left with a permanent neurologic deficit, which included an inability to talk and paralysis of the right side of her body. A computed tomographic (CT) scan of her head revealed an intracerebral hemorrhage in the left cerebral hemisphere. How does this case illustrate important principles of clinical pharmacology?

2. A 35-year-old woman was near the end of her third trimester of pregnancy when she developed a urinary tract infection. Her physician made the proper diagnosis, and asked her about any past drug reactions. She mentioned that she had received a sulfa drug several years before to treat a urinary tract infection, and several days later had developed a total body erythematous rash. Not wanting to repeat this experience, her physician prescribed Bactrim™, one double-strength tablet to be taken twice daily for 10 days.

After 2 days on this medication, she began to develop a red rash all over her body. The next day, she developed a fever and the rash worsened rapidly. The drug was stopped, but the rash progressed until much of her skin peeled off (a severe exfoliative erythroderma). She was hospitalized and treated as if she had a severe total body burn.

Discuss her case with reference to the scientific basis of treatment and individualization of treatment.

ANSWERS

1. Prescribing drugs rationally is essential to minimize toxicity and maximize efficacy. There are several key steps you should run through in your mind as you develop a therapeutic plan for each of your patients.

First, do your best to establish a diagnosis. In this case, the patient had developed a mild acute urticarial reaction to hymenoptera venom. She did not develop a more severe (anaphylactic) reaction, since there was no manifestation of angioedema, bronchospasm, hypotension, or shock. Thus, any necessary treatment should be "mild," since her condition was "mild."

Second, understand the pathophysiology of the illness. You have already made the primary distinction that needs to be made in this case with your diagnosis above. The mild allergic urticaria seen in this patient was primarily caused by the release of histamine from mast cells in the skin. Other vasoactive autacoids may also be released, but histamine seems to be the primary mediator.

The third step is to pick the best drug, based on your understanding of the disease pathophysiology. This is where the physician went wrong, either because he made the wrong diagnosis of anaphylactic shock (in which case epinephrine would be the drug of choice), or because be did not understand that this patient's illness is best treated with a histamine-receptor blocking drug such as diphenhydramine. Epinephrine was not indicated for this mild reaction.

The fourth step is to individualize the treatment plan. We already know that epinephrine was not the drug of choice. However, the physician who prescribed epinephrine did not realize that this particular patient would react to epinephrine in a peculiar way. Epinephrine activates both alpha-adrenergic and beta-adrenergic receptors. At therapeutic doses, the alpha-receptor–mediated vasoconstrictor effect predominates, but the blood pressure does not increase so dramatically because of activation of beta-adrenergic receptors that cause vasodilation. Since the patient was receiving a beta-receptor blocking drug (for unclear reasons!), the unopposed alpha-agonist effect of epinephrine caused a hypertensive crisis with tragic results.

Fifth, the physician should recognize that the administration of any drug is really a therapeutic experiment, and appropriate endpoints for the experiment must be chosen. If diphenhydramine had been given, appropriate endpoints to follow would have been a resolution of the urticaria and the development of somnolence. If epinephrine were given, one would want to follow pulse, blood pressure, tremor, or other signs.

Sixth and finally, the physician should make a "contract" with the patient. He must not only follow the patient with close supervision during this therapeutic encounter (or misadventure), but he must help with other related problems down the road. For example, he may give advice concerning education about the self-administration of an antihistamine after a bee sting. He may wish to discontinue the propranolol under supervision, especially if there was no clear indication for it. If the propranolol must be continued, he may wish to order a bracelet for the patient, warning of drug interactions with propranolol. In other words, the "contract" with the patient only begins when a drug is ordered or given—it doesn't end with the prescription.

2. Sulfonamides are capable of eliciting numerous allergic skin reactions. The total body erythematous rash was entirely consistent with sulfonamide sensitization, and it correctly served as a warning to the physician that sulfonamides should be scrupulously avoided in this patient because an even more serious reaction might be precipitated with the next exposure.

Bactrim™ is the trade name for a fixed ratio combination of sulfamethoxazole (a sulfa drug) and trimethoprim. It is an excellent drug for most urinary tract infections, but it should not be used in patients with a history of sulfonamide sensitivity. In this patient, it produced a prompt and very severe exfoliative reaction.

Not only should this patient's treatment have taken account of her prior reaction to sulfa drugs, but her therapeutic plan should have recognized that her pregnancy was late in the third trimester. At that time, it is unwise to administer a sulfa drug because of the danger of inducing a syndrome called kernicterus in the neonate. Ampicillin would be a good drug to use in this situation, since she has no allergy to penicillins, and penicillins are considered antibiotics of choice at any time during pregnancy because of their excellent safety record for both mother and fetus.

In short, the therapeutic plan for any patient should take into account the features that make that patient unique—in this case, the patient's pregnancy and prior reaction to sulfa drugs. Other patients may have other relevant conditions, such as renal failure, liver disease, heart failure, asthma, drug allergies, pharmacogenetic factors, concomitant drug therapy, or age. Your consideration of all of these features as you prepare your therapeutic plan—your deliberate synthesis of clinical medicine and basic pharmacology—is at the core of the practice of rational therapeutics, and at the core of the discipline of clinical pharmacology.

Your therapeutic plan must be firmly based on scientific principles and clinical data, with adjustments as needed to take into account those features that make your patient unique. A "cookbook" approach that treats all patients with a certain disease similarly will often result in suboptimal or even dangerous therapy. Individualizing therapy offers a better chance of maximizing efficacy and minimizing toxicity—the goal of a rational approach to therapeutics.